Let Your Life Flow

First published in 2002 in the United Kingdom by
The C.W. Daniel Company Limited
1 Church Path, Saffron Walden,
Essex, CB10 1JP, United Kingdom

ISBN 0 85207 357 7

Produced in association with Book Production Consultants plc,
25-27 High Street, Chesterton, Cambridge, CB4 1ND.
Designed by Marion Hughston.
Printed and bound by Cromwell Press Ltd, Trowbridge, England.

Alex Maunder

Let Your Life Flow

THE PHYSICAL, PSYCHOLOGICAL

AND SPIRITUAL BENEFITS

OF THE ALEXANDER TECHNIQUE

Illustrated by Lucy Guenot
Index compiled by Lyn Greenwood

SAFFRON WALDEN

THE C.W. DANIEL COMPANY

Let Your Life Flow

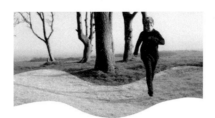

CONTENTS

Dedicated to my wife, Andrea, for all her love and support,
and to my four beautiful children. Also to my ever-living guru,
Paramahansa Yogananda, for his inspiration, love and immortal wisdom.

"Everyone has self-limiting idiosyncrasies. These were not put into your nature
by God, but were created by you. These are what you must change -
by remembering that these habits, peculiar to your nature,
are nothing but manifestations of your own thoughts."
(Paramahansa Yogananda)

ACKNOWLEDGEMENTS

I would like to express my thanks to all my Alexander colleagues, in particular to Misha Magidov, Illana Machover, David Clarke, Graham Griffiths and Harpa Gudmundsolottir. To Lucy Guenot for her wonderful drawings, to Doug Baillie for the cover photograph, to Sarah Maunder for her photographic skills and to my publisher Ian Miller for all his support and encouragement and for his great sense of humour.

Photographic acknowledgements: The photographs of FM Alexander are the copyright of The Society of Teachers of the Alexander Technique. Child at play and the Mountains in the Mist were photographed and the copyright held by Sarah Maunder. The two photographs of Pharaoh Kafre, the gold death mask of Pharaoh Tutankhamen, and Pharaoh Menkaure with two wives are the copyright of the Egyptian National Museum, Cairo. Woodland Light was photographed by, and is the copyright of, Leonard Smith. Let your voice be free was photographed and is the copyright of Rosalind Simon.

Let Your Life Flow

Foreword

WRITER'S BLOCK

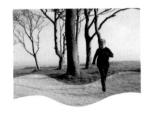

I have been meaning to write this book for a long time, its been one of my projects that I never seem to get around to. I manage to write the book plan, but the book itself gets put off. There are delays from the publisher's side (which I gratefully accept) there are always more important things to do and suspiciously the weeks lengthen into months and years and there is still no sign of *"The Book"*.

Until one day I wake up and realise - I'm suffering from writers block. This isn't right. I mean I'm meant to be showing people how the Alexander Technique can be a way to health, happiness, mental clarity and success and I can't even help myself to write a book! It's a bit embarrassing really.

So I repeat "Let the neck be free, to let the head go forward and up, to let the back lengthen and widen" endlessly to myself, like a mantra, until I begin to feel quite comfortable and less worried and even less inclined to write *The Book*. I begin to feel quite hopeless.

I think it's just lack of willpower - I should get up earlier, get more focused, drink more tea or coffee and work longer hours, but still the aim of my willpower fails to hit its objective, as if an invisible force field were deflecting it. I begin to realise that there is an internal saboteur at work, a part of the personality that wishes to keep me feeling stuck and full of fear. Unless and until I work with reconciling and reintegrating this part of myself all my efforts will be in vain.

So I retire to a quiet room to work on myself. I know that this routine will take about 20 minutes of my time but that I will come away feeling immeasurably refreshed and revitalised. The whole day will be different, with a clearer mental focus and energy flow. At the end of the day more will get done and the quality of the work will have been higher than if I had just forced myself to work towards my goal, ignoring all the signs of resistance and the blocked energy flow in my mind and body.

Sitting comfortably in a well-supported arm chair I decide to work with myself as a psycho-physical being. I need to stop being so goal orientated and work with understanding and transforming the physical and emotional blockages before I can get more energy and more mental focus. So I take time to focus on my physical sensations first of all and how that is making me feel. The most immediate sensation I notice is that my body feels very hard and tight, constricted with fear. It is almost as if I feel powerless to move or act and my worst fear is that I will never be able to escape from this terrible place.

What do these words and physical sensations link to? What does this mean in the story of my life? It links to a feeling of disempowerment, of never having been able to set clear goals and to achieve them. I can make an enthusiastic start, but somehow I lack the stamina to complete. I often feel a sense of inner wobbliness, which means that I can easily be swayed and persuaded by powerful figures in my family and immediate environment - thus losing sight of my original intentions. There is fear as well, a fear of action that is linked to a fear of making mistakes. It is better to sit here and to do nothing than to go forward and to risk making a mistake. I feel terribly stuck.

Paying attention to my body language has helped me to define the problem, but what can I do to break out of this constricting, fear-filled hole ? I sit down and I use the next two steps of the Three-Step Technique that will be described later on in this book, of opening myself through the power of "directions" to the greater potentialities that exist as my inner world connects with the outer spheres of the surrounding Cosmos. As I reach a state of calmness and interiorisation several subtle bodily shifts and releases begin to take place and my consciousness clarifies itself. I feel that I have regained a wonderful sense of spaciousness in my body, of lightness, and in that space there is now room for a free flow of energy and intelligence. At the same time I shift into a more relaxed and confident mood with a vibrant sense of self worth. My attitude shifts to a sense of - OK, I'll give it my best shot and if I make it fine, if not, I'm still an OK person.

Several other thoughts rise strongly to the surface of my consciousness.

• If we want to have a real sense of self-worth, we have to feel it in our bodies as a positive, expansive feeling. There has to be that golden glow within, a real physical sensation of expansion and upliftment.

• It is painful to admit responsibility for our mistakes, to see the part that we have played in a co-created process. It is easier to go into victim mode and to blame others 100% for our suffering, thus making them the persecutors. However, if we do have the courage to take responsibility for our part of the mess that we are in then it empowers us - because we can change that part of our behaviour in the here and now. Taking responsibility enables us to grow.

• The past is irrelevant, it doesn't matter anymore. The only thing that matters is what we have learnt from our mistakes.

• Victim consciousness and the body language that goes with it can be transformed by an inner energy flow that is strong, balanced and vibrant. The posture is carried by the inner vitality and the world responds to a positive body language in a miraculously different way.

Feeling calm and clear I focus my attention on the bodily shifts that had taken place and ask myself what they mean for me. I feel completely different in several key areas. Several words come to mind that describe the shift. I write them down:

"My heart is uplifted, I feel joyful
(a strong, overpowering sense of joy)

My hands and feet are tingling
I'm ready to get on with things

My breathing is soft and deep
I feel purposeful and grounded

My mind is clear and focused
I will follow my star."

Now I can start to write. *Alex, Let your Book Flow.*

Chapter 1

INTRODUCTION

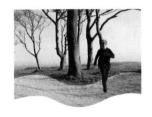

This is a book about the Alexander Technique. Its aim is to show how the mind, body and emotions can work as one happy, harmonious whole and how you can effortlessly and smoothly achieve all your objectives in life. Alexander was one of the first people to actively work with the psycho-physical unity of himself and then, later, of his students. He was a pioneer in what is now a very obvious concept: that your mind influences the body and that your body posture and gesture will affect the way you are thinking and feeling.

We need to understand his Technique in terms of the materialistic, scientific world view that prevailed at the end of the Victorian era, as the 19th century drew to a close and humanity entered that era of ever-accelerating technological change known as the 20th century. This Newtonian, mechanistic world view is essentially materialistic because it seeks to understand the world by breaking things down into their component parts so that we know how they work. It then uses that knowledge of the causal laws of Nature as a power in order to improve our physical health or environmental comfort as a path to happiness.

It seems quite a good idea, doesn't it? Until you realise that this view of the world is always going to be dealing with parts and not wholes, dealing with symptoms rather than causes and viewing human beings as material objects rather than as spiritual beings. A doctor or a scientist who is trained in this way runs the danger of becoming overspecialised, of knowing more and more about less and less, until he or she knows everything about nothing! Scientific knowledge runs into the danger of becoming terribly specialised and fragmented. We have not trained our scientists and doctors to think how *systems function as a whole,* nor to think how these different holistic systems (eg, human beings) interact with each other and move towards their common evolutionary purpose, which gives an overarching spiritual perspective.

Alexander was one of the first people to react against the prevailing materialistic world view. Through painful experience he came to realise that his problems were not just 'physical' problems that could be solved through drugs, surgery or the application of more will-power and mental focus. He couldn't just pursue his ambitions and hope that the problem would go away. No, his 'problem' was actually a messenger in disguise sent to teach him something important about his life. Alexander learnt to work from his *whole self* back to the specific part that was causing him problems. He found that he had to work with his state of mind first, as a primary consideration, before he could heal (literally, make whole) his persistent physical problem.

This is the first book that seeks to explain the subtlety of Alexander's Technique in clear, up-to-date language and concepts. This book also shows for the first time how the basic principles that Alexander discovered can be used to process physical, mental and emotional disharmony (that leads to dis-ease) and to bring them all back into harmony with our higher purpose in life. Up till now the Alexander world has tended to ignore emotional problems that students bring with them and to say, "That is not our field. Please go and seek counselling or psychotherapy." But this is immediately creating an artificial split between mind and body and contradicts Alexander's basic philosophical view that we are a *psycho-physical unity.* This book aims to show Alexander teachers, trainers and students that we already have the tools, we already have the principles that work across all levels of the psyche and that can lead to a total and radical transformation of the self. What is obviously needed is training and experience, and the quantum leap in thinking that can take the Alexander Technique out of a restricted little pigeon-hole that says, "Alexander Technique: good for releasing muscular tension patterns and improves your posture; much used by actors and musicians." No, the Alexander Technique is much, much more than this. There are universal spiritual principles here that will allow each person to be guided by their inner-soul wisdom and to be led out of restriction into a consciousness of peace, harmony and joy.

The old paradigms, the old Newtonian, mechanistic world view causes problems, lots of problems. It leads to a narrow, egotistical attitude and the sort of body structure - uptight, constricted, fearful and top-heavy - that keeps people trapped in that space. It leads to disaster, because both individually and collectively it leads to a completely selfish and self-seeking attitude. Egotism on a collective level leads to ecological exploitation of the planet. On a political level it leads to power politics (rather than the politics of consensus). And on the economic level it leads to selfishness that concentrates wealth in the hands of a few countries and leaves many others in terrible poverty. But it cannot continue for ever, because it breaks so many spiritual laws and causes so much tension that it will break down under the weight of its own top-heavy structure. The Alexander Technique has nothing to say on these sorts of issues, but it has very much to offer on a practical level. No solutions can be imposed from the top downwards; they have to grow from the base upwards. It is only as each individual person works on themselves, to transform their *psycho-physical selves,* their reactions and behaviour, only as each individual takes responsibility for their self-improvement can we have a better society and a better planet. Personal and planetary evolution go hand in hand.

So what does *psycho-physical unity* mean? It is actually hard to imagine what the full implications are of this little phrase if you have not experienced them. One person might say, "I take care of my body; I go to the gym regularly; I have a massage every now and then because I know that the state of my body will affect my mental focus and efficiency at work." Fair enough. That is one attitude and it is a start (certainly much better than going home at night, eating a pizza take-away and crashing out in front of the TV), but there is still a division between mind and body. This person spends periods of time taking care of his body in the gym and other periods of time being mentally focused and efficient at work. This is not psycho-physical *unity*. There is still a division even though that person is trying to give equal importance to both body and mind as equal partners at different times.

Another person might do Yoga or Tai Chi every week and say, "I know what psycho-physical unity is, I can really feel how my mind and body work as a unity as I flow into these movements or hold these asana positions at full stretch." I would reply, "Great! You really appear to be 'in the flow' during your classes, but look at your posture during the tea break! Collapsed in your seat, sprawled over a cushion, hunched up over your tea, you have lost it all the minute the class stopped. There is no connection between what you learn in your class and your daily posture and movements. I'm not trying to knock Yoga, but there is still a great contrast between the periods of practice and the rest of your week."

A third person might have regular Alexander Technique lessons. They would say, "Of course I know what psycho-physical means. I have read all the Alexander books; I have wonderful posture and smooth-flowing movements that I maintain during daily activities. I maintain a sense of connection between mind and body by continuous practice of the Technique throughout the day. I feel up and light, full of energy. Of course I know what psycho-physical means." I would reply, "OK, you came really close, but the circle is still not complete because you have neglected your emotions. What about those emotional outbursts that you have from time to time where some little thing has pressed one of your buttons and you appear to have lost all self-control for a period of time? Is that a proper way to behave, and what has happened to the quality of your psycho-physical unity at these times? The serene detachment and awareness have gone and you appear to be bound up in your emotional reactions and overwhelmed by your problems of the moment. That is not true psycho-physical unity because the emotions have got out of control and have affected the harmony of the whole. You were flying high, but then you lost it."

Psycho implies not only the mind but the emotions as well, and physical implies not only the body but the emotional memories, the traumas that are locked into our bodies. E-motion is the flow of energy and cellular changes that surge through the body as a result of our thoughts and reactions to circumstances. You cannot maintain the harmony of the psycho-physical whole if you ignore the effect of emotions. They are there and they have to be acknowledged and appropriately expressed or processed in some way. You ignore emotions at your peril because they never just go away; emotions are energy and that energy, if it is not expressed appropriately, will get lodged and stored in the body memory. Every time the right button gets pressed they will be released in a powerful flood, seemingly from nowhere. Psycho-physical unity means being able to express and process your stored-up emotional memories.

Many people go for regular counselling or psychotherapy sessions, where they seek to understand their emotional reactions (or lack of them) and the root causes of their psychological problems. But they often fail to see how they are ignoring their physical side, so that they may be perpetuating their problems and situations by their body language in the present moment of time. This is the psychological work without any physical input. So clients may learn to understand themselves better in an analytical way, but they often fail to learn how to change themselves. Sometimes, even, their therapist may comment on their posture, gesture, facial expression or quality of eye contact. This is good practice and helps to increase awareness and increase the emotional expression of the client. But it is still not what I would call truly *psycho-physical work* because clients are not taught how to change their body language; so therefore the subconscious compulsion to repeat the old behaviour pattern still remains. Also it has not put the client in contact with the guidance of their body wisdom so they lack a higher intuitive perspective from which to view their problems.

Now, however, modern scientific research is backing up the empirical findings of therapists and teachers who have been trying to work in a truly psycho-physical way. Modern science recognises that the human body functions holistically. We have an intelligent body where every cell has the potential to communicate with every other cell, and every cell is intelligent. Thinking and memory are not confined only to the brain. We have a body memory as well. Recently I attended a very exciting lecture given by Prof. Allan Schore from the Department of Psychiatry & Behavioural Sciences at the University of California (Los Angeles Medical School). His work is on the neurobiology of emotional development.

Using the most modern scanning techniques and testing for minute traces of chemical particles, he and his colleagues have been able to monitor the brain development of infants. Their research findings are truly fascinating. When a traumatic event happens, eg, the mother frowns and speaks aggressively to the child, the memory of that event is stored simultaneously in *two separate memory banks* in both the left and the right brain hemispheres. As is well known, the left brain hemisphere (which controls the right side of the body) is the logical and rational side of the brain. So a factual memory of the event - the frowning face, the tone of voice and what was said - is recorded there. However, the right brain hemisphere, which is the symbolic, holistic, artistic and emotional side of the brain, records a separate emotional memory of the event. This emotional memory is recorded as the feeling of the stomach clenching and churning with fear, the ribcage tightening, the heart palpitating and the breathing getting fast and shallow. The emotion is fear, but it is connected with a whole series of physical sensations in the body.

Now, these two memories are connected but separate, and they can trigger each other off. So in later life when this infant grows up, and maybe now he works in an office, one day his boss frowns at him and starts to heavily criticise a report that he has written for the firm. He suddenly feels overwhelmed by a feeling of fear and insecurity; one of his buttons has been pressed. His stomach starts churning, his heart starts palpitating and he cannot breathe properly. He may either feel completely put down and incompetent, or he may feel a great, childish rage towards his autocratic and domineering boss. Mostly, because he is in an inferior position, this feeling would be repressed, and he would go home thinking, "What a terrible day I had at the office today; I hate my boss." Now for me the phrase *psycho-physical unity* would mean someone who is aware and could understand and process what was going on both mentally and emotionally as well as physically, and use the higher wisdom of their body to find an attitude shift and so come back to a place of perfect peace and harmony within themselves.

Psycho-physical unity means more than an awareness of how the body and mind interact; it means coming into contact with our higher intuitive wisdom which I call our *Body Wisdom.* Through a holistic awareness of our psycho-physical unity we can reach a higher level of intuitive awareness and inner guidance. The myths and fairy tales of the world abound with stories that describe this process in a symbolic form. The hero or heroine is on a difficult quest and has to make a journey of some sort in pursuit of something precious that the evil one has stolen from them - which is basically their consciousness of wholeness and integrity of being. They encounter many trials and fearsome enemies on the way, and at some stage they meet the form of an uncouth and rather stupid-seeming animal (or animals). And yet when they take their minds or egos off their great quest for a moment to befriend this seemingly stupid and insignificant beast (representing their body-consciousness), and pay attention to it and love it for what it is, then an amazing transformation takes place, and the beast is transformed into a shining prince, or it displays some incredibly useful strength or quality of feeling or intelligence that then helps the aspirant to attain the triumphant conclusion of their quest. This apparently magical transformation is the shift that takes place when we follow the universal principles, and the whole point is that we are never strong enough to do it alone, relying only on the limited concepts of the mind and ego. But, if we pay attention to what our bodies have to say, to those energies and parts of us that we have judged harshly and denied, then we have the chance to transform them and reintegrate them in a rediscovered sense of wholeness and integrity of being, so that we shall experience the fulfilment of our quest.

Chapter 2

THE
ALEXANDER STORY

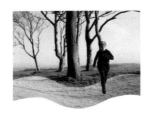

Alexander was an Australian actor, a Shakespearean reciter who did one-man shows and had built up a rather successful practice for himself in Melbourne at the end of the last century. He had studied music and drama and loved the theatre, but his promising career was soon threatened by a tendency to hoarseness and respiratory trouble during performances. He went to various doctors, but they were unable to help him as there were no obvious physical causes for his disability. But, being a man of lively intelligence and indomitable will-power, he decided that the only thing left to do was to cure himself. This was the start of his journey of self-discovery.

The first step that he undertook was to reason things out, as he was essentially an intellectual and reasoning type. If his voice was getting hoarse during recitation but not at other times, this must be a result of something specific he was doing when he was reciting on stage, but not at other times. Quite logically for him then, the start of the healing process must consist of finding out exactly what it was he was doing wrong and to observe the problem objectively. To do this effectively he set up a system of three mirrors so that he could observe every part of his head, neck and throat when he was in the process of recitation. After a period of painstaking observation he realised that he was doing three things: he stiffened his neck (thus pulling the back of his head down); he depressed his larynx unduly (by tightening muscles deep inside his throat, thus pulling his chin in); and he gasped as he sucked in breath.

Now these were minuscule movements that he observed in himself, millimetres rather than centimetres, but two things became apparent to him immediately. Firstly, he hadn't felt this happening within himself (a phenomenon he came to term 'faulty sensory appreciation'). And, secondly, his muscular activity didn't appear to be under the direct control of his conscious reasoning mind - because when he ordered his muscles to relax and stop tensing they refused to obey him; in fact the tension seemed to increase. It was obvious therefore that the direct approach wouldn't work, but what alternative was there? It took Alexander several years to work out the answer to this problem. Others who have come later can now benefit from his work and learn the Technique from a qualified teacher, but Alexander had to work out these principles all by himself, and this took an enormous length of time, patience and will-power. He was not, however, one of life's victims, but an overcomer who recognised that, no matter the problem, its mere existence gave rise to the possibility of an answer; and he decided to keep on trying until he found it.

THE THREE PRINCIPLES OF SELF-TRANSFORMATION

The first thing Alexander tried to do was to define his problem objectively, to examine himself and his inner processes as if he were a perfectly detached observer. But defining his problem also meant perceiving it in its wider context and not just as an apparently random set of muscular reactions. Thus he also began to notice that, in addition to pulling his chin in, depressing his larynx, and pulling his head back and down, he was also lifting his chest, narrowing his back, shortening his structure and failing to 'take hold of the floor with his feet' - that is to say, ground himself. What is more important still is that he also came to the vitally important conclusion that his mental attitude was also at fault.

Alexander was over-ambitious. He wanted to get to the top as quickly as possible, to gain recognition and applause, and to be known as one of the best actors or directors in Melbourne. As a result of this ambition he was trying too hard, and this in turn led to over-tensing and quite literally getting in the way of himself, effectively blocking the full expression of his rich inner potential. Now Alexander made these observations and connections in the same way a scientist might - logically and meticulously he proposed a hypothesis, experimented on himself and observed the precise results of his experimentation in a three-way-mirror system. He realised that he had unreliable sensory appreciation, so that what he felt was not necessarily what was really happening. This problem of unreliable sensory appreciation can of course be overcome once a person has spent time and effort to develop themselves through the use of the Alexander Technique.

He also made one further vital observation and that was that this whole psycho-physical reaction pattern which he had observed was not just something that happened when he got up on stage and started to recite, it was actually present at all times (though in a milder form) a habitual way of being that he had falsely identified with so that when he got up to recite it would just be automatically triggered off, and dominate any attempt he might be making to behave differently. So the implications of all this were very far-reaching: if he wished to change his habitual way of being (his habitual 'use of himself', as he termed it) it would have to be at all times, not just the few important times when he needed it. He would have to work not only with the physical manifestation but also with the mental and emotional attitude behind it. And the final test, the ultimate proof of his state of being would be shown to him by his body - but it would have to be the whole body-mind experience that enabled him to relax any particular set of muscles.

Alexander now knew very clearly what the physical component of his problem was: he was tensing his throat and neck muscles, pulling his head back and down in relation to his spinal column, and he also recognised what the mental and emotional component of the problem was: he was too much of an achiever, a doer, an 'end-gainer', as he termed it. Yet, try as he might, he could not rectify the fault by direct means. The more he tried to stick his head forward and up (which was the opposite of his habit pattern and therefore the logically correct solution), the more he seemed to end up with a stiff neck and a hoarse voice at the end of the day. It all seemed merely to exacerbate the problem.

If the direct way was not going to work then Alexander had to find an indirect way, and being a man of great perseverance he kept at it until he had found a workable way around this problem. Firstly, he had objectively defined his problem: he knew what was happening in his body but he couldn't work out how to stop it happening, because every time he put himself in that position (starting to recite) his old, instinctive, reaction pattern took over. But if you can't stop something happening *you can at least stop trying to stop it happening* - stop fighting it; stop fearing it; create space and acceptance by being non-resistant to the whole situation. Just allow yourself to *observe* rather than thinking that you have to do something about the situation. So his second step was to do absolutely nothing at all. This moment of pause, this quiet moment of keeping calm within himself, he termed 'inhibition', which is not to be confused with the Freudian use of the term, and it proved to be the key that would unlock the door for him. Alexander's reasoning was impeccable. He realised that his power of free choice appeared to be greatly limited because, once he was caught up in that situation, the power of habit appeared to be much stronger than the wishes of his conscious, reasoning mind. But he did have one clear area of choice open to him, and that was the power to say YES or NO to the whole situation before he got involved in it: YES, I am attached to my desire and tied into doing something about the whole situation; or, NO, I do not want to do anything at all.

Now this was a very important place to have reached because it allowed his ego to step out of the picture for a moment to create a space, a creative silence where the cloud of unknowing could enter and work its transformative magic. You see, he really didn't know what the answer was. Everything that he knew came from the past, which was just the accumulated pattern of his previous thoughts, feelings and actions, and the experiences resulting from these. Every time the conscious, reasoning mind (ego) had tried to suggest a solution to him it had failed. He had tried holding his head this way and that way, getting hold of the floor with his feet, regulating his breathing, projecting his voice in a different way, doing this and doing that, and none of it had worked. Because his way of doing came from the past, and was the result of his past experiences. He had not known the answer in the past - if he had he would not now be in the mess he was in - so why would the continuation of past patterns of misuse suddenly bring him liberation and success in the future? Something new was going to have to arise in the present, creative moment, the eternal NOW; and if it was to be truly new then by definition he would have no idea, no preconception, of what it might be. He was going to have to stop doing and start being; he was going to have to allow forces to work through him rather than thinking that he knew it all already.

So he just put a full stop to all doing, all striving and just waited in a state of creative awareness. He later coined the phrase, "When you stop doing the wrong thing, the right thing will happen all by itself."

There is no outer activity here, but there is a state of very clear inner focus on what is; the over-tensed muscles, the irregular breath, the emotional states of tension, fear, anger or ambition - whatever it is - just accept it, look at it, and be true to it, because that is what is happening in the moment. It is not the way it will always be, but it is the way it is at the moment, and that is our starting point in the process of transformation, the raw material that we have to work with. And then a very curious thing starts to happen: by acceptance and by looking at things or people calmly and without judgement, without trying to do anything about it, we create space, and by creating space we allow things to unfold and develop in harmony with the pattern of their inner being. Our body posture doesn't like being continually tensed and shortened. People don't like being continually judged and put down. These are all unnatural states that are indicative of a lack of harmony and balance, and if we just allow enough neutral space for it to be, there appears to be a force in the cosmos that is striving towards peace and harmony, and will redress the balance.

In one sense Alexander was opening himself up to the wisdom of his own body, or those forces that could act through his body and guide him. Inwardly he was saying,

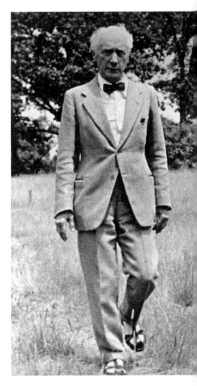

FM Alexander Walking

As a result of his technique Alexander was able to maintain a beautifully poised alignment and a sense of balanced release in all activities. Notice how the relaxation extends even into his fingertips.

"I'm not sure any more, so you show me. I'm going to give up ordering, preconceiving, theorising and being so sure that I know, and I'm going to say, 'Well, actually, I don't know anything any more, so please, you show me.'" Rather than chasing the answer all the time, why not give it time and space to come to you? Let the answer emerge from the problem itself. Because, as is portrayed in the Yin/Yang symbol, the seed of the solution is already contained in the problem, and if you do not meet with immediate success, don't be discouraged, because it is always darkest just before the dawn. Patience, waiting, and an inner stillness become the keys to the whole situation.

Now a most remarkable thing can happen when you attain this quality of attunement and clear awareness: things start to shift. A process of inner organic growth can take place and new directions emerge that can point the way forward. It all happens without us doing anything; it is the true process of non-doing. So this is the third stage of Alexander's work, the third principle of self-transformation: when something begins to grow from inside as energy is liberated from all the old habitual tensions, blockages and limitations. Fear dissolves away and the mind leaps over the shadow of its former preconceptions, experiencing freedom.

To take Alexander's specific case, he had a tendency to depress his larynx at the back of his throat and to shorten the muscles at the back of his neck, thus pulling his head back and down onto his spinal column. When he had effectively mastered the technique of coming back to himself and keeping very still, quiet and aligned within himself - a technique which he termed 'inhibiting' his habitual responses or, refusing to react - then he found that a process of organic growth and release could begin to take place within his body.

The ball of tension that had been concentrated in his neck and throat area began to dissolve, to melt away, and as it did so he found his jaw releasing forward and his head releasing upward (from above the atlanto-occipital joint); at the same time the whole of his vertebral column began to release and lengthen right down to the coccyx. There was also a feeling of the whole back widening across the shoulders, ribcage and pelvis. Thus, from his specific problem area, there was a shift into a general pattern of release. Once having experienced this shift he then formulated his now famous affirmation, *"Let the neck be free, to let the head go forward and up, to let the back lengthen and widen,"* which was his way of describing his release into freedom. By repeating this affirmation to himself it was also a way of actualising this new, positive shift when under difficult and stressful conditions. Needless to say each individual is unique and will have a different pattern of tension because they have had a different life story, but wherever our specific muscular tension patterns are located, these principles will work (if we let them) because they represent the shift from tension into freedom. These are universal healing principles.

It is necessary to be receptive, to allow things to happen, to be open and allow the counterbalancing qualities to flow through to us, but we have to have faith in the process and allow things to happen in perfect trust and confidence. This quality of letting things happen appears to be central to the Alexander Technique and all forms of healing work or self-transformation. One thing that Alexander found particularly helpful for this whole process was if he remained connected with the cosmos through mental 'directions' projected outwards in space. The most important of these are Up, which is a projection of the spinal column up to infinity through the top of the skull, and Down, which is a grounding through the pelvis and the soles of the feet in a line which drops through to the centre of the earth. The third most important direction is to allow the shoulders and shoulder blades to drop downwards and then to widen. If these mental directions are projected effectively, they produce great calmness and stillness within the body, because we are getting connected with the cosmos mentally and energetically, but there is absolutely no sense of striving or straining. We should never try to be bigger or different from what we are; there is always 100 per cent acceptance of ourselves and our situation at this point in time. But we are waiting, and watching, and giving permission for something new to happen - when the time is right.

There are so many different systems and forms of therapy around nowadays, but I for one always want to know: what is the key element here in this process of self-transformation, what is the golden key, that will finally unlock the door? Very often when you penetrate through to the core of it you will find that it is actually a nothingness, a stillness, a quietness, a calmness and a waiting. If you are spiritually inclined you could sum it up in the words, "Be still and know that I am God." Or if you are humanistically inclined you could just describe it as a state of perfect inner balance and alignment, getting in touch with your own limitless inner potential. It actually doesn't matter how you describe it. What matters is whether you are able to experience it or not. It is something that can be practised again and again every day in a whole variety of situations, because these principles work, and they work on every level - physical, mental, emotional and spiritual. If we are feeling emotionally unbalanced and out of sorts for whatever reason, we can work with ourselves in exactly the same way, but we need the time and space in order to be able to take our own emotional processes seriously.

If you want to learn this process then you need to be able to go into a quiet room and shut the door so that you can be alone for 10 or 15 minutes. You will need to sit down and start talking kindly to yourself, saying something like, "OK, what's the problem? What's my body trying to tell me? What am I really upset about?" (step one). Key to this is realising of course that a disharmony will be reflected on all levels simultaneously so it is very instructive *to be aware of the pure body feeling of it first* because this often helps the intuitive mind to gain direct perception of the true cause of the problem. Step two: the creative 'waiting without preconceptions' as you give 'directions' through the length of the spine and out of the top of the head allows a shift to take place. This is pure 'non-doing'. The final stage, step three, is making a cognitive link so that you can understand *how* these physical shifts make you feel different mentally and emotionally. Certain words or phrases will suggest themselves to your mind and from these, just like Alexander did, you can construct a positive affirmation that will help you to maintain this new state of being in your work, relationships, goal-setting, etc.

The longer I practise this work, on myself and with students, the more the beauty and simplicity of it appeals to me. Step one - looking at yourself honestly and taking responsibility, non-judgementally, for what has happened - that is your part of the work and it is essential. Step two consists of getting yourself out of the way, but really 100 per cent out of the way, and realising that you don't have to fight your battles. Step three is then taking what you have learnt and putting it into practice in your daily life - because if it only remains at the level of a mental insight then it hasn't really changed anything at all! There are so many problems that you feel stuck with, and you have fought so hard and so long, but they are still there. Finally the penny drops - the way of direct confrontation doesn't work, so why not try the subtle, the indirect approach? Hand over your problem, surrender it completely, get so in tune that it actually doesn't seem to matter any more whether or not you are suffering from this dreadful, insoluble affliction. Hand it over, don't fight it any more, and in that acceptance and attunement comes the downflow of counterbalancing qualities that brings release and healing. In some inexplicable way the whole problem just seems to melt away and it will be lifted off you. It is then up to you to go out into the world and be a different person.

It really seems as if there is a force that is striving to restore peace and harmony in our lives, and in all the conditions that confront us. Whatever qualities you need to restore harmony, be they on the physical, mental, emotional or spiritual plane, will be given so that you are then able to experience health, wealth, love and perfect self-expression. Whether you are stuck with an unbearable relationship, insoluble problem or seemingly incurable disease in your life, it is basically an indication of a lack of balance, a lack of harmony. By using the Alexander principles, or any other effective healing techniques, you will be able to restore balance and harmony to your life, by opening the channel for the downflow of all that is good and true and beautiful.

Every time someone appears to have been struck down by some apparently incurable disease, their career stopped short, their prospects ruined, and yet they cure themselves from within, with no help from the medical profession - every time this happens, you should study their story carefully and honour the indomitable spirit within them. But let us also realise that whilst you can learn from them, you also have to make these principles your own, a part of your experience and your own inner life. And in that difficult process there is also a very real sense of rediscovering these principles for yourself. Once you have made them your own in a very real and intimate sense, what you have made your own on the inner levels, nobody can ever take away from you. So when this happens you also have to honour yourself as a pioneer and overcomer, and you are then empowered to pass these principles on to others who are also in need.

Chapter 3

THE
TYRANNY OF HABITS

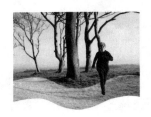

The essence of the Alexander Technique is about how to change our habit patterns. Habits exercise a tyrannical hold on our character and therefore on our destiny. The Alexander Technique gives us a very effective tool for change. As one of my Alexander Technique students said when I asked him how he felt different as a result of his Alexander Technique lesson, "I am not my habit patterns. I am OK." When you contact your core through the Alexander Technique there is a realisation of peace, calmness and serenity.

When trying to change you have to realise that it is the whole bundle of physical, mental and emotional habit patterns that you are up against. At first, as Alexander thought, it might appear to be only an annoying physical habit pattern that you are seemingly blocked by. But then the realisation dawns that there are also deeply ingrained mental and emotional habits that have to be changed. *The key point to remember, however, is that while there is a physical pattern of release which is the same for everybody, there is a*

Child at Play

Young children display a superb sense of balance and alignment before the onset of bad postural habits in later life. Notice the natural lengthening along the spine and the freedom of the neck, which is maintained even when jumping.

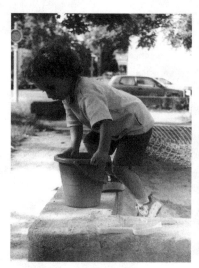
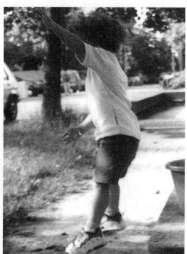

psychological pattern which is unique. This is a point of fundamental significance because, eg, my habit of hunching my shoulders might look the same as your habit of hunching your shoulders, and through 'directions' we both might be able to drop them, release downwards with gravity, open and widen the shoulders. However the *psychological cause* of my original tension pattern and what it means for me to experience that sense of openness when it releases is completely different from what it means for you. We are two unique human beings with unique experiences and life stories.

First we need to understand how the muscles work, and then we can examine more fully how the mind and emotions habitually interact with them in a stimulus/response model.

HOW MUSCLES WORK

There are two types of muscles in the body: voluntary and involuntary. You are supposed to have control of your voluntary muscles, but as Alexander discovered, due to the power of habit, you have much less control over these muscles than you would like to think. Voluntary muscles are also called skeletal muscles because they are attached to the bones of the body, and due to their power of contraction they are able to bring about movement around a joint. Muscles can only cause movement by their ability to contract. There is no propelling force in their ability to lengthen, which is merely a relaxation. And your choice as a conscious human being is always a simple YES/NO - do I wish this particular set of muscles to contract or do I wish to relax it by not contracting? When you wish to move, a muscle will contract because of a stimulus from the central nervous system. In the spinal cord of the central nervous system are thousands of nerve cells called motor neurons. Each of these nerve cells connects to several muscle fibres by means of a long nerve fibre, so that when you decide to do something - such as lift up a cup of tea - your decision to make this movement is transmitted through the nervous system to the appropriate muscles, and you can act through your ability to make those muscles contract. But please note, you can never do anything to *force* a muscle to lengthen again. You might think that you can force the body to be taller or to widen across the shoulders, but this is always at the cost of extra tension elsewhere in the system, and after 5 or 10 minutes you will tire of the strain and collapse again. The only real solution is to turn off the switch as it were and stop wishing to contract the over-tensed muscles that are causing the problem in the first place. Whether the muscle fibres then release to their full length or not is something that will be discussed in more detail later on. Due to the power of habit, or of mental and emotional tension elsewhere in the system, the muscle fibres may not release fully even when you consciously ask them to do so.

In addition to understanding how the motor nervous system works, it is helpful to understand how the sensory nervous system works. This system gives the brain and nervous system information about movement and thus gives you your kinaesthetic sense. There are nerve endings attached to every muscle fibre which send sensory information to the central nervous system. These are called sensory neurons and are located in the joints, muscles and tendons of the body. They respond to any movement, stretch or contraction by sending information along the nerve fibres to the sensory nerve cells situated in the spinal cord. From there the information is transmitted to the brain. Highly jointed structures such as the neck, wrists and ankles will be able to transmit a lot of information. The neck in particular is very sensitively tuned to the slightest movement, unless the muscles of the neck have become too tight and therefore minimally responsive to the delicate movements of the head in relation to the rest of the body. When the neck is fixed, due to over-tensed muscles, the amount of sensory information you can receive is reduced. In addition to the sensory neurons, you have a balance mechanism situated in the inner ear which is an important part of this kinaesthetic awareness.

UNRELIABLE SENSORY APPRECIATION

There is a drawback to the way in which the whole muscular and nervous systems interact and Alexander called it 'unreliable sensory appreciation'. This is due to the fact that the mind is a bit like a computer: very busy with lots of important things to think about, so that many routine actions, eg, stretching out your arm to pick up a cup of tea, are done in a habitual way, on automatic pilot, as it were; and this very clever computer-like mind simply says to the nervous system: "Just tell me when something goes wrong, tell me when something different happens. If not, just carry on and do it the way you've always done it, OK?" Now, if you pick up your cup with chronically over-tensed shoulder muscles or finger and wrist joints, then that information would have been conveyed to the brain via the sensory neurons at the beginning; but when this becomes a habitual fixed state then there is no new information for the brain to receive and register. It has become the 'normal' state; nothing has changed and the brain isn't receiving any new information. This then accounts for the fact that someone can have chronically over-tensed neck and shoulder muscles and yet feel completely relaxed and normal.

So what options do you have for re-educating the body, mind and nervous system so enabling you to break out of this closed circuit? The first option would appear to be to re-sensitise the body by allowing chronically shortened muscles to lengthen again during the course of an Alexander Technique lesson, thus giving yourself the experience of breaking habitual boundaries and being able to reactivate the sensory nervous system. This happens during hands-on work (it can also happen as a result of increased receptivity and being prepared to go from the known to the unknown as described elsewhere in this book). Visualisation and persuasion (rather than force) have a key role to play in this. So this is the first option: have Alexander Technique lessons which will release the over-tensed muscles and reactivate the sensory nervous system.

The second option would appear to be to bring the conscious, reasoning mind into operation so that you become aware of yourself as 'thinking in activity'. In other words you turn off the automatic pilot and decide to bring conscious awareness into all stages of your movements as an aid to this process of re-education. You can train yourself to make movements slowly and consciously, being aware of exactly what muscles you need for that particular movement and what muscles you can leave relaxed. You can be aware of balance, both within the body as a whole and within a particular body part, as the muscles subtly shift in relation to each other and as your weight gets redistributed in the course of movement through space and time. The key point to remember is that the mind is engaged in conscious awareness of the movement during the whole time, rather than putting it on automatic pilot.

The third and final option is to cultivate the opposite good habit with which you wish to replace your previous bad habit, and then to repeat it often enough until it replaces the old tendency. Now obviously this must be divided up into subtle stages, because, if you were to launch straight into doing what you thought to be the 'correct' thing, you would merely end up on automatic pilot again - caught in the same old patterns as before, however good your intentions might have been. If, however, you give up even the intention of doing it, let alone the actual physical activity, and merely visualise the most balanced, easy and natural way of carrying out that action, then you have a chance of re-educating the body and nervous system and eventually you will actually be able to put into practice what you have visualised as a perfect image in your mind.

Alexander's solution was a combination of these approaches. He decided to emphasise thinking rather than feeling, because he knew that (in the beginning at least) trying to feel if he was doing something right or wrong was not going to give him reliable feedback on what was actually happening to his body. So incorporating thinking and actually ignoring what he was feeling became an important part of his system. He also decided to make an important distinction between means and ends, so that instead of trying his hardest to get things right, he would be aware instead of the things that he was doing wrong, the tension patterns that were getting in his way and actually preventing him from achieving his aim. In other words, he gave all his attention to not pulling his head back and down, to not shortening his neck muscles, emphasising the process of change rather than its results. Alexander called this paying attention to the 'means whereby' rather than 'end-gaining'. So instead of trying to *do* the right thing, he experimented with thinking the right thing, by maintaining thought projections, and *doing* nothing. It was by working in this way that he came to recognise the inseparable nature of mind and body, which were in his words, a 'psycho-physical unity'. Biofeedback machines that can register the level of muscular tension in the body have since demonstrated precisely these discoveries made by Alexander at the turn of the last century through self-observation.

The Stimulus/Reaction Model

Alexander realised that the core of his problem lay in being caught up in habitual reaction patterns that felt right, that felt comfortable, even when they were in fact wrong and damaging. After a long period of study he came to the conclusion that there is a tiny point of freedom that lies between the stimulus and the compulsion to respond. You are all aware of certain areas of your lives where there is a trigger that leads to a rapid and almost automatic response. I say 'almost' because you do have this tiny point of freedom where the possibility exists to initiate a new response pattern, acting from conscious choice, guided by your higher wisdom that takes you into unfamiliar territory and gives you the possibility of real growth and change.

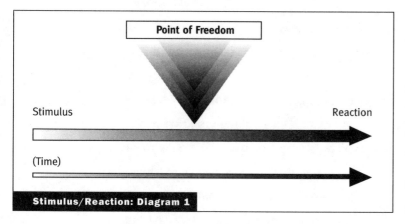

Stimulus/Reaction: Diagram 1

Let's look at this diagrammatically.

As you can see from Diagram 1, Time runs along the horizontal axis. There is a specific stimulus at the start; perhaps you

are asked to give a presentation in front of a group of people, or perhaps a woman says something to you in a particular tone of voice, with a particular look that just happens to remind you of your mother. Depending on what your particular fears or subconscious memory patterns might be, this could be a stimulus to a major reaction pattern. Wham! Your button has been pressed and you are into a major emotional upheaval. The point of freedom has been passed without you ever having known that it was there. It is so tiny that you missed it.

This is a very familiar theme now; there are no end of psychological self-help books published that are trying to help you to become aware of what your 'buttons' are, how you are reacting automatically and how you can change that reaction pattern if you don't like it. You can recognise your 'buttons' for yourself. The key indication that a button has been pressed is the intensity of the emotional reaction pattern and the way you become totally bound up in the whole thing. There is no space left for the detached observer because you get sucked in by the intensity of your emotions and the compulsion of a painful yet strangely familiar energy.

There are no end of psychotherapy groups that you can join to explain to a sympathetic listening group how you feel trapped in a particular situation, or a particular relationship, and how the pattern just goes on repeating and repeating without the power or the possibility of change. Well, the group may be listening sympathetically, but they don't believe everything you say, especially not the bit about, "I don't have the power to change." It is just that at some level *you are choosing* not to change, you are choosing to remain stuck, because it feels safe in that same old place, and you recreate your past experiences again and again. Freud talked of the neurotic 'compulsion to repeat', Alexander talked of the 'automatic habitual response', and it's the same thing: you can be aware that you are stuck, you can even (on the rational, conscious level) dislike the feeling of being stuck, and yet you are still unable to break free.

Well, over 100 years ago Alexander had news for the world, especially for people who felt they were caught in a psycho-physical habit pattern. There is a way out, and it comes from recognising that there is a 'point of freedom' - it's just so small, and you can be travelling so fast, that you don't see it coming. Once you have passed that point it is very difficult to get back there because you are generally so caught up in your emotional reactions that it is difficult to disentangle yourself and view the situation objectively. Alexander's advice was always to first stop and say "No" to the situation. Stay in balance and refuse to react habitually. Go inside to contact the power of your deep inner core and from that place you can decide what you

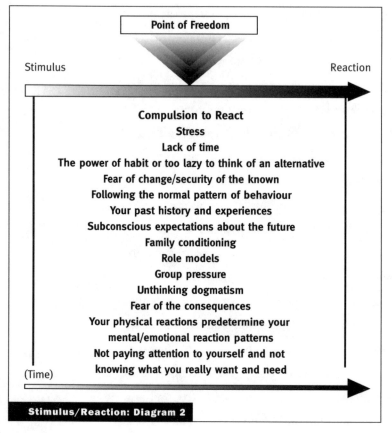

Point of Freedom

Stimulus

Reaction

Compulsion to React
Stress
Lack of time
The power of habit or too lazy to think of an alternative
Fear of change/security of the known
Following the normal pattern of behaviour
Your past history and experiences
Subconscious expectations about the future
Family conditioning
Role models
Group pressure
Unthinking dogmatism
Fear of the consequences
Your physical reactions predetermine your mental/emotional reaction patterns
Not paying attention to yourself and not knowing what you really want and need

(Time)

Stimulus/Reaction: Diagram 2

want or what is right for you at this particular moment in time. This may be a fairly quick process for some people, but for others it can require a lot of time. So much so that you may even need to say, "I need more time. I'm not sure about that at the moment but I will get back to you when I know for sure." That's OK because it's all part of the process of making a good decision and choosing what you want from a place of freedom rather than being forced to react by subconscious habit patterns.

You can look at the factors that tend to force you to react automatically, and then at the interventions that can help you to widen the point of freedom, to create more space and time so that you are acting out of free choice rather than compulsion. In Diagram 2, I have listed some of the major factors that can compel an unthinking reaction.

These are all fairly predictable factors that contribute towards us living unthinking, fearful and stressed-out lives. Many people complain about stress; more and more complain about lack of time, as if the world is somehow speeding up and there are now less than 24 hours in a day. The power of habit and the power of environment impede your ability to make free choices from the core of your being - deep down inside where you know what is right. The mind can justify anything; you can rationalise anything when in reality your main motivation might be fear of change and clinging to the security of the known. Due to your subconscious expectations or early conditioning you can actually be under a compulsion to continually recreate your past experiences, again and again and again - ad nauseam. This is the main work in any therapy and it is slow, hard work that can take many years. But the brilliance of Alexander's insight was that you are psycho-physical beings and as such your

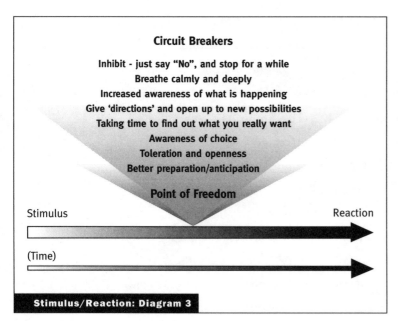

Circuit Breakers

Inhibit - just say "No", and stop for a while
Breathe calmly and deeply
Increased awareness of what is happening
Give 'directions' and open up to new possibilities
Taking time to find out what you really want
Awareness of choice
Toleration and openness
Better preparation/anticipation

Point of Freedom

Stimulus   Reaction

(Time)

Stimulus/Reaction: Diagram 3

automatic physical reaction patterns in any situation can actually predetermine how you are going to feel and what you are going to think. You can become completely trapped, for a time at least, in a closed circle.

Now you need to look at the interventions that can help us to widen the point of freedom and allow us to choose rather than just react. Take a look at Diagram 3.

The most obvious thing that you can do to give yourself more space and time and widen the crucial point of freedom is to just stop and say "No" - refuse to react and refuse to make any decision for a while. A rushed decision is a bad decision and one that you will invariably regret later on. It is better to make no decision rather than the wrong decision! So just pause and give yourself time to think. This is like the pause that a good actor introduces at a crucial part of his speech, the 'think about it' pause. Or it may be like the familiar request to sleep on an important decision. Or it may be the realisation that you just don't know what you really want and that you need more time to find out. You do not have to live life at a frantic pace the whole time. Nature is constantly exhibiting the principle of ebb and flow, flowing through the different seasons, and life too can have its moments of not knowing and introspection rather than only instant answers and constant activity. It is OK not to know and you can remain calmly poised at the point of freedom, uncommitted but free, rather than rushing into a decision or ill-considered action that will be binding later on.

Breathing deeply three times is a great aid to help you remain in this space of non-reactive calmness. You need space and time to increase your awareness of what is really going on and it can be a whole tangled web of factors that all interrelate. One of Alexander's greatest insights was that we are psycho-physical beings, and our physical reaction patterns can actually predetermine our mental/emotional reactions. There is no freedom here - just an automatic response. For example, I had one student who, for reasons going back into her childhood, lacked confidence, and standing up for herself and getting what she wanted was associated with feelings of 'waves in her stomach', tensed shoulders, and feeling very unsure of herself, emotionally unloved and left out in the cold. In later life, making decisions against the opposition of others was a nightmare for her. With the help of Alexander lessons she learnt to breathe deeply, to refuse to react for a while whilst giving 'directions' (which will be explained more fully in Chapter 4), which helped to relax her muscular tension pattern and open up her posture. We had introduced a circuit breaker into the system. By changing her physical reactions she was then able to think more clearly and calmly and as she became aware of what was really happening, she said, "I feel calmer and more independent. I trust myself more; it really doesn't matter what others think; they are more in the background; it's *my decision.*" So new possibilities opened up for the future.

It is so important to find out what you really want. Some people are so clear that they just know instantly, others take longer to find out. Due to previous conditioning your head may be saying one thing, but your heart or your gut-level response may be something completely different. It can take time to find out what you really want and that is OK because it will give you an awareness of the true range of choices available to you.

There is no freedom without a choice. There have to be at least two options (or even three or more) to choose from before you can say, *I am free - I have a choice!* If you are reacting from a place of compulsion then you have only one option and no choice at all. This is a point of fundamental importance if you wish to understand the philosophy that underlies the Alexander Technique. It is this point that changes it from being a mere posture therapy into being a psycho-physical technique that restores your freedom to take responsibility for your life and to live as a truly free human being. It is not for nothing that one of Alexander's books was entitled *Man's Supreme Inheritance.*

Diagrammatically instead of having only one stimulus and then only one automatic reaction you now have one stimulus and two or even three options to choose from. You have created a gap and then have used the point of freedom to become aware of your different options. You now have the opportunity to find out which one you really want. Now you can choose and move forward in life. Only by working with the psycho-physical reality of the 'Self' can you bring about the deep-rooted character change that will enable you to move forwards in your life.

As you can see in Diagram 4, by inhibiting your automatic response and saying "No", first you have enlarged the point of freedom into an area of freedom and two new options have been discovered: Reactions 2 and 3. They existed all the

time but you just
didn't have the space
and the calmness to
be able to spot them.
If you can say "No"
and remain calm for
long enough it is
possible to make a
rational choice about
the best option and to
take responsibility for
it. This is crucial,

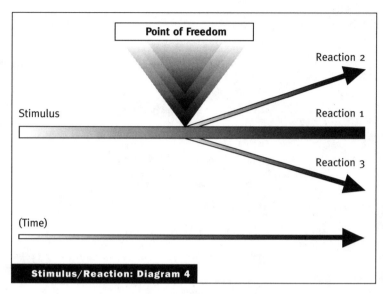

Stimulus/Reaction: Diagram 4

because it makes a huge difference if you feel that you are being
coerced into something rather than making a free choice. You may
feel that even though you may not like it you still wish to choose the
original course of action (Reaction 1) of your own free will, and that
you will see it through to the end. The fact of the matter is still the
same: you may still be choosing Reaction 1, but the attitude of mind
is completely different.

It is all about responsibility and choice. Most people do not take
responsibility for the situation they find themselves in. "I am in this
relationship but I have nowhere else to go and I feel trapped. I have
to stay." To that I would reply: Rubbish! You are not choosing to be
in the relationship but you have a subconscious compulsion to set up
a situation where you will feel trapped because that is what you are
used to. Another client might say, "I wish I could get rid of this
aching back, it's making my life a misery." I would be forced to reply:
What is the misery in your life that you cannot express in any other
way except through your back? The minute you can actually take

responsibility for your life and realise that *at some level you are actually causing it* then you can choose not to do that, and then choose an alternative course of action or mode of expression. But, as Alexander realised, first you have to raise your level of consciousness so that you can become aware of what you are actually doing to yourself. So awareness is the first step and then you can take responsibility for what you are doing to yourself, for the pain that you are causing yourself. Then follows the desire to change and the decision to change.

What does the word responsibility really mean? It really comes from response-ability, ie, the ability to respond to a situation. But as our earlier discussion about Alexander's philosophy, the stimulus/response model and the point of freedom all show, in order to respond adequately to life's demands you have to have at least two choices of response. Then you can choose freely, and having chosen as a free human being you will then have the ability, the stamina and the commitment to maintain that response over time. That is my definition of a responsible human being. In a society that is gravely lacking in ethical decision-making and responsible behaviour at all levels of political and economic leadership, any form of training or any philosophy in action that helps people to arrive at the point of freedom, and to make responsible decisions from that point, has to be a vast improvement on the present chaotic and immoral situation.

As you can see from the preceding discussion of Alexander's stimulus/reaction model, if you are tied into the past and you only have one way of reacting then you will feel trapped and history will go on repeating itself (because Life is trying to teach you a lesson and you are just not getting it!). If you wish to attain freedom and take control of your destiny then you have to know how to reach the point of freedom and have choices. It is as simple as that, you can switch from victim mode to conqueror mode. The only way to control the world is from the inside by mastery over yourself and over the compulsion of habits. Someone once said, "It is not the things that happen to us *but our reactions to them* that determine what we are like as human beings." And character is destiny, because a different character will attract different relationships and different circumstances to itself in the fullness of time.

Chapter 4

THE BASICS OF THE ALEXANDER TECHNIQUE

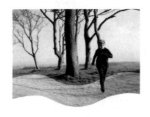

A basic definition of the Alexander Technique would be that *it enables you to perform each movement or maintain a posture with the minimum amount of tension.* This makes sense, doesn't it? Many people want to be more efficient, to achieve more by doing less, and maybe the basic motivation is inherent laziness. I have a fundamental belief that for every problem there is a solution, and not just any solution, but a beautiful, elegant and simple solution. Scientists researching into the laws of nature are beginning to suspect that there is an intelligence behind all of creation, because when searching for a theory or an equation to explain natural phenomena, it is always the simplest and most elegant theory that fits the data and expresses the laws of nature. Well, Alexander found a simple and beautiful explanation for the law governing efficient movement and posture and he called it 'primary control'. This is a central integrating factor, a key to the efficient functioning of the whole organism. Alexander observed this phenomenon in animals and in humans; he observed this most of all in himself through the use of three mirrors. Put very simply, this law of primary control says that if the head is freely balanced on top of the spinal column at the atlanto-occipital joint (ie, if it is not being pulled back and down onto the neck and shoulders) then there is an integrating flow and poise throughout the whole organism, so that the head leads and the body can follow. Alexander's theory of primary control is simple, elegant and, above all, practical. He proved that it worked on himself, and it has worked for thousands of Alexander Technique students all over the world.

Alexander would always poke fun at learned academics, professors of physiology and anatomy who were top men in their own field and full of theoretical knowledge, but some of them suffered from the most terribly misaligned and contorted posture. It was obvious that they had a tremendous amount of specialised knowledge about nerves, muscles and the skeleton, but it was all theoretical knowledge and they had not discovered the integrating principle of the primary control.

It is the same when you go to a medical doctor or physiotherapist and, for example, complain of lower back pain and a misaligned pelvis. They will obviously try to correct the problem there through massage or ultrasound or even cortisone injections, applying their specialised knowledge; but they will not stop to consider if perhaps over-tension in the neck muscles or a misalignment of the head on top of the spinal column could be causing the problem. They are not trained to look at the system as a functioning whole. Can the neck muscles affect the pelvis, or can the misalignment of the pelvis affect the neck? An Alexander teacher would say, "Yes, of course it can!" Because we are trained to look at the whole, the way it all fits together and the central integrating function of the primary control. Actually, an Alexander Technique teacher is rather unconcerned with the specific symptom at its point of manifestation because we are more concerned with a holistic view of the whole system and the way the individual parts fit into that. If the primary control can be brought into operation and the general alignment and energy flow of the body improved, then through the law of balance and harmony the specific problem will be healed. It will just disappear. The root meaning of the word heal is 'to make whole'.

The concept of primary control is subtle; it takes time and the direct experience of many Alexander Technique lessons to really understand it. It is an elusive and slippery concept that keeps eluding the grasping intellect. It is basic to the Alexander Technique, but there are certain preconditions that need to be in place before primary control can manifest itself. These are the four main pillars of the Alexander Technique: balance, breathing, directions and mental calmness. Once these four main pillars are in place you are in a much better position to allow the primary control to be experienced.

Now Alexander wanted this 'improved use' of the whole organism to be integrated into daily life. This isn't just theoretical knowledge; you don't just read about this and then forget about it. This is applied knowledge. This is philosophy in action. The sense of ease and flow that result from the integration of the Alexander Technique with your daily life is truly remarkable. There is a sense of connection with your Self at the deepest level and intention flows seamlessly into activity in movements that seem to involve the whole of the body. The sense of tension and separation into several conflicting body parts has disappeared. This is replaced by a sense of integration and flow.

THE FOUR MAIN PILLARS OF THE ALEXANDER TECHNIQUE: BALANCE, BREATHING, DIRECTIONS AND MENTAL CALMNESS.

Balance

The Alexander Technique is designed to inhibit our stressful reactions to life, reducing muscular tension and anxiety levels so that we can relax and achieve more by doing less. It is about balance: physical, mental, emotional and spiritual balance. An absolute precondition of this is for the body to be physically in balance, and by this I mean a very precise balance line in the body where the skeletal system is in balance and the muscular system hangs loosely around the skeleton with just the right amount of muscle tone to keep the body erect but without excessive tension. If you are even a few millimetres out of your balance line there is already excessive tension in the system. Students of the Technique learn how to re-establish a sense of conscious balance in the body, to develop a calm sense of inner poise and how to support a healthy posture. Movements become freer and more flowing; the body feels integrated and you live more in the moment with a heightened sense of awareness and enjoyment of life.

There is one vital question you can always ask yourself at any time of the day, whatever you are doing: "Am I standing or sitting consciously and aware of my balance line or am I standing or sitting habitually, holding myself in a certain position because that is just the way I always do it?" The implications for your sense of body awareness and vitality are very different in each of these two possibilities. It is like day and night.

Developing an accurate, conscious sense of balance is absolutely vital if we wish to sit, stand and walk in the Alexander way. If you observe yourself closely in a mirror, sideways on, you will notice that you are probably not standing or walking with a balanced, upright posture. A neutral line of balance in the body (see Figure 1) would pass from the crown of the head, through the atlanto-occipital joint (the joint where the skull balances on top of the spinal column), down through the shoulders, the centre of gravity in the

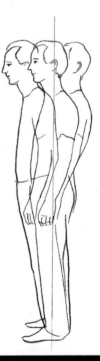

Figure 1

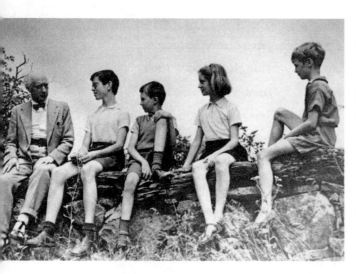

FM Alexander Sitting with a Group of Children

Look how beautifully balanced these children are sitting on a stone wall in the company of Alexander. If you wish to improve your children's posture remember: they will follow your example and not your words.

pelvis, the hip joint, the knee joint and straight down through the ankle and heel and into the ground. So there is a line that joins a point on the crown of your head and passes down through your body and into your heels. Look at the balance line in Figure 1 and let your eye become familiar with the design idea of the body.

Using the help of the mirror just check out your line of balance; notice if it appears to be too far forwards (most people are), or backwards. Now allow yourself to sway gently and slowly backwards and forwards; feel the whole line of your body moving from your ankle joints as you sway like a tree in the wind. Feel how you come too far forwards and you have to tense your muscles in the lower back to keep upright; notice how when you go too far backwards you have to tense your stomach muscles to stop yourself losing your balance. Be aware also of what is happening in the soles of your feet, how the weight distribution changes. As you sway forwards more weight comes onto the balls of your feet, and as you sway backwards more weight goes onto the heel until you reach that dangerous place where the toes start to come off the ground and you can feel yourself on the edge of falling over backwards. So you are playing with different possibilities, feeling the range of movement that is possible. Now begin to make the movements smaller and begin to notice more the point when you actually feel that you are in your balance line. For a fleeting moment you have it and then you lose it again. When you are in your balance line you may notice that there is more upthrust from the heels, up the legs, up the pelvis, up the spine, and that because the spine feels stronger the head can balance in a different way on top of the spinal column. You will notice that the weight distribution in the soles of your feet has changed so that there is now slightly more weight in your heels than in the balls of your feet. Make the movements smaller and smaller until you finally come to rest in what feels to you like a neutral balanced position. Keep breathing, don't try to 'hold' this position, just enjoy the sense of having attained conscious balance.

Another simple and effective way of working with balance is to contrast the line of the spine being extended upwards through the crown of the head, with the downward weight of all the relaxed muscles being pulled to the earth by the force of gravity. Starting of course with the throat and neck muscles, continue with releasing the chest, stomach, arms, back, buttocks, legs and feet muscles - all the way down. The effect is rather like hanging clothes on a hanger, except in this case the muscles are being draped over the framework of the skeleton. In this variation the upward thrust of the spine and head is balanced exactly against the grounding effect caused by the muscles drooping downwards. This might appear to be very easy and simple in theory, and it is, but it takes constant practice to achieve mastery of balance.

So this is an exercise that you can start off doing at home with the aid of a mirror (or perhaps a shop window when you are out shopping), but as you get more experienced at this you get to trust your inner kinaesthetic sense as this becomes more reliable, and you can get to read your body posture from the weight distribution in the soles of your feet. So you can do this at various odd points of the day: waiting for a bus or a tube; waiting at a supermarket checkout; standing up drinking a cup of tea during your tea break; the possibilities are endless. And the benefits in terms of lightness, ease of movement and increased energy supply are well worth the small amount of effort. Each time you make a small effort to change your postural habit patterns with an exercise like this the benefits are cumulative.

As you work with this balance exercise you will gradually come to realise that we not only have a line of balance, but we also have a 'centre' which is the centre of gravity of the body, located in the middle of the pelvis about two finger widths below the belly button. The Japanese call this the 'Hara' and attribute tremendous importance to it. Certainly, if you can locate this centre you are able to regenerate very quickly and you can work from a centre of calm and stability. As you work with this simple balance exercise you may become aware, or your Alexander Technique teacher may point out to you, that you are unduly arching your lower back, exaggerating the hollow and tilting the pelvis so that the base of the spine is pulled backwards and upwards. This puts undue pressure on the vertebrae in that area - causing strain and backache - and it also blocks the flow of energy through the

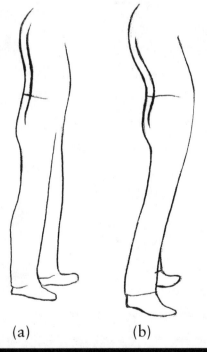

(a)   (b)

Figure 2

spine. Observe the two contrasting shapes of the lower back and spine in Figure 2.

As you work with the balance exercise it is imperative to release this tension in the lower back if you wish to connect with the power of your Hara, your centre of gravity. What is needed is for the back to lengthen and the buttocks to drop down and round so that you can then experience true grounding through your legs. This is not a 'doing' - ie, trying to position the pelvis in a certain way - it is a very subtle and effortless sense of 'releasing' the excessive muscular tension, which then allows the spine to lengthen and the pelvis to swing into its correct alignment relative to the balance line and the spine.

If you have difficulty doing this on your own (and most people do!) then it is important to have personal Alexander Technique lessons so that your teacher can give you the hands-on experience of what it is like to release through the power of directions (see the later section in this chapter on 'directions'). This gives you the experience of moving from alignment (a) to alignment (b) in Figure 2, but with an effortless sense of ease and lightness. The secret that will be transmitted through the hands of the teacher and then later taught to you verbally is *how to give 'directions' to first widen across the width of the pelvis and then to lengthen down the length of the leg* which is the most effective way to release the tension at the back of the pelvis.

Once the spine can be properly grounded in the pelvis, it is possible for the spine to lengthen upwards, thus freeing up the weight of the chest and shoulders and the balance of the head on top of the spinal column, and to continue the sense of the pelvis widening and the legs releasing at the hip joint, thus giving a sense of greater space and power in the pelvis. By bringing your personal centre of gravity into balance and harmony with the Earth's gravitational pull you are able to experience a sense of release and sustainment, which at first is a purely physical sensation, but later on you begin to deepen your awareness of its psychological and spiritual implications. Then you can come to experience how Hara (your centre of gravity) is actually a power centre - as the Japanese well know.

Finally, creating this inner balance within the body gives you the paradoxical experience that by doing less you are achieving more. By relaxing downwards you are generating an upward thrust, a new sense of vitality in the spine and skeletal system, as well as increased tone in the musculature. You learn to embrace and harmonise the Yin and Yang within your consciousness, and to regenerate yourself from the inexhaustible source of Hara, your power centre.

Breathing

Next breathing, because breath is the bridge that links the mind to the body. When you are emotionally upset, the rate of respiration increases; and when you are calm and serene, the rate of respiration decreases significantly. As we are psycho-physical beings the one influences the other in a continuous feedback loop, so that either through mental focus and detachment, or through learning some sort of breathing technique you can bring the system back to a state of stable equilibrium.

Alexander's main concern was with acting and voice projection when on stage. Any actor needs to get enough air to support his voice during a long Shakespearean speech, as Alexander well knew! The timing of the pause and the timing of the breath is vital. The quality of the voice is also important because there needs to be a sense of power and resonance which can carry into the furthest corners of the theatre. The power for this sound comes from a resonance in the belly rather than the high, tight sound that comes from a constricted throat. To get the breath flowing easily and smoothly is the essential foundation of voice work.

To improve your breathing you first have to understand the mechanism involved in breathing. The main muscles that produce the pump-like movement of your breathing are the diaphragm and the intercostal muscles between the ribs. The bony structure of the ribcage itself is there to protect the heart and lungs. The lungs are the organs of breathing and are like two large air sacks positioned on either side of your heart. They are surrounded by the 12 pairs of ribs which make up the ribcage. These are all attached to the thoracic spine at the back; but the two lower ribs, the so-called 'floating ribs', are not attached to the sternum in the front. The other attached ribs are spring-loaded, ie, they want to expand again once they have been compressed. There is an actual physical power of expansion in those ribs, so much so that if you cut the ligaments that attach them to the sternum they would literally fly open! So you see, there is already a mechanical advantage built into the movement of the expanding ribcage. The two 'floating ribs' at the bottom of the ribcage, being unattached, are capable of a greater sidewards expansion than the rest of the ribcage. They can float sidewards like the wings of a bird during inhalation. This is an essential part of Alexander breathing.

The rhythmic movement of breathing is driven by the diaphragm. This is a an umbrella-shaped piece of muscle that fits below the lungs and on top of the stomach, liver and spleen. It acts like a pump in that when you inhale, the diaphragm muscle contracts, pulling down the floor of the diaphragm and thus increasing the size of the thoracic cavity above it. When you exhale the diaphragm relaxes and moves back to its resting position, thus decreasing the size of the chest cavity. This regular movement is continuously operating the breathing mechanism, massaging the organs around it, and aiding the healthy function of the circulation and digestion.

It is impossible to engage in the Alexander Technique without first calming the breathing. This calms the mind, soothes the emotions and brings you into a deeper contact with your core Self. The whole nervous system has to slow down so that you are able to calmly observe and make connections rather than be restless and nervous. When relaxing on the floor in the semi-supine, or at odd times during the day, it is good to practise some Alexander breathing. The first thing to notice is that the breath is actually flowing the opposite way from what people normally think. You may think that you breathe in through your mouth and that air fills the top lobes of the lungs before moving on down. You may also think that the opposite happens as you exhale, that you empty the lungs from the bottom up. If this is what you feel to be happening then you are probably forcing the breath in using the muscles at the top of the chest, which are the wrong muscles to use, and you have completely the wrong pattern of breathing. Due to the pump action of the diaphragm you actually need to visualise and feel the air flowing up the body as you inhale, filling the lower lobes of the lungs first and then the upper lobes last. This should be a long slow breath. During exhalation you need to visualise the air

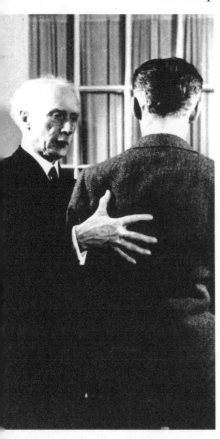

FM Alexander Working on a Pupil

Through his hands Alexander has built up an energetic contact with his pupil. The depth of his mental focus is shown in the serenity of his facial expression and the calmness of his breath.

emptying from the top of the lungs back down the body towards your diaphragm and abdomen. In this type of breathing it feels as if the air enters and leaves from your abdomen (which is the area centred just below your belly button).

The important point in Alexander breathing is that the lungs need to be emptied completely during exhalation. If there is any effort used, and sometimes there does need to be a bit of effort at the start of a breathing exercise, the effort should go into ensuring that all the air is fully expelled from the lungs, especially the bottom lobes. Then you have to let go and allow the air to flow in all by itself, without any sense of will-power or muscular effort being used. The point is that if all the air has been fully expelled as the ribcage contracts and the diaphragm relaxes and returns to its top position then a partial vacuum has been created in the lungs and atmospheric pressure outside will push the air back into the lungs, through the nose or mouth, in order to equalise the pressure outside and inside the ribcage. Once you have breathed out fully, atmospheric pressure will do its stuff and refill your lungs with air. Leave all anxiety behind, trust that the air will flow from a high-pressure to a low-pressure zone, and realise that no one has yet managed to kill themselves by forgetting to breathe. Practise this a few times now.

If you have practised this correctly, ie, without any sense of effort or will on the inhalation, then you may have noticed a steady, calm, continuous quality to the in-breath. This comes from the sense of 'non-doing', from the standpoint of being a detached observer, watching quietly as the laws of the universe work to sustain your being. However, you may also have noticed all the things you are doing to prevent this.

Firstly, incorrect posture. If the shoulders are rounded and the front of the chest is caved in then you have greatly reduced your lung capacity. No matter how long you practise you will never achieve a sense of effortless ease in your breathing, it is impossible to improve your breathing until you first improve your postural alignment and allow the shoulders to release and open out. So posture and breathing work together, and both are basic to the work of self-improvement.

Secondly, unnecessary muscular tension. As explained earlier there is a natural elasticity to the ribs; once you have created a vacuum through a full out-breath the ribs want to expand and fill with fresh air. If this isn't happening the question is what are you doing to prevent it? As you try to practise non-doing on the inhalation, if you pay careful attention, you may well notice where you are holding. Are your stomach muscles too tense? Are the ribs held? Is the sternum (the bone at the front of the ribcage) too tight? In the Alexander Technique we are very much concerned with spotting these unnecessary patterns of muscular tension and releasing them through awareness and 'directions'. It would be a waste of effort to try and force the breath more against the resistance of this muscular holding. By releasing the tension you can achieve more with less effort. Some of the key areas to be aware of are: to release the stomach muscles; to give directions to *allow* a widening across the back of the ribcage; and to give directions to *allow* a widening across the top of the chest and to lighten the sternum rather than let it collapse downwards.

The key quality, however, is learning how to empty the lungs completely and allow the in-breath to flow in without any sense of will-power or effort. To get to that space, however, you need to let go of anxiety, let go of worries, let go of fear and resentment, and just watch the breath. At first you need to expel all the air on exhalation, but after a while you don't even need to do that. Be calmly detached as you allow the breath to flow in and out by itself. There is an ocean of air surrounding you and each breath is a little wave that ebbs and flows from that ocean. But the ocean is always there to support you. As you watch the waves come and go you get a sense of peace, calmness and serenity. The mind is clear and focused, the body is relaxed. Gradually the realisation comes - I am not breathing, I am supported by the ocean of breath and 'It' breathes me. What a wonderful sense of release and sustainment comes from this realisation. The respiration rate slows down, the heart slows down. As you continue to watch the breath you may even start to notice small pauses between the breaths, you will feel that you do not need to breathe immediately, that it is quite comfortable to exist for a time without breath. Go ahead and enjoy the breathless state without any sense of fear or strain. This is the basis of all meditation techniques.

This is also the basis of all voice work. If you want a strong, calm voice that resonates from the abdomen, if you want to gain and hold your audience's attention, then you have to learn mastery of the breath and mastery of the pause. There are natural pauses in a text or presentation, where something important has been said and you want the message to sink in. To the speaker a pause of several seconds can seem an eternity of time. Their underlying anxiety is that they don't want to appear stupid or as if they have forgotten what to say. So the tendency is to rush and you lose your audience's interest because you appear to be anxious and going too fast. If you have said something important and you want the message to sink in, then you have to allow a pause at the appropriate moment, and the message is - think about it! In that pause you need to employ your Alexander breathing. This means that you make sure you have exhaled fully, then you allow the breath to flow in by itself without any sense of effort until the lungs are comfortably full. This will take several seconds but you are giving your audience time to think and you are giving yourself time to recharge from within. By the quality of your attention as you *allow the breath to flow in* you are calming and centring yourself. There is a power that then radiates out from your centre and holds the attention of other people in the room. When you next speak the audience becomes magnetised by the calmness and strength that resonates in your voice. That power can then be expressed in many modes but there is a fascinating magnetic attraction that goes beyond words.

Directions

What is a 'direction'? In his writings, Alexander talks of sending 'directions' or 'orders' for muscles to release and to lengthen, eg, "Allow the neck to be free." He was projecting these orders in order to counterbalance his tendency to tense his neck muscles and pull his head backwards and down.

His famous and original formulation of directions was:

> "Allow the neck to be free,
>
> *to let* the head go forward and up,
>
> *to let* the back lengthen and widen."

The original emphasis was on the word *let,* but, human nature being what it is, beginners will tend to pick up on the words "go forward and up" and "lengthen and widen" and try to *do* it - which is completely counter-productive. You cannot *do* it because that is just adding more muscular tension to an over-tensed situation and you will also be trying to put your head into a preconceived position which is based on your habitual feelings of rightness and, therefore, is bound to be wrong. We are all such doers that it takes a lot of self-observation in order to be able to spot that tendency to 'do' and turn it around, so that we learn the art of 'letting', being more receptive, being a non-doer and letting things happen. Which is what Alexander's little word *let* is all about.

In all his writings he always stresses that directions are combined with inhibition. This is absolutely crucial because otherwise the tendency to 'do' will always creep in. In other words you have to stop and say, "No" and continue to project your directions for the new use of yourself. There must be no desire to change anything (for example, let me just adjust the position of my shoulders here, or readjust the angle of my pelvis there, in order to make things better, etc). The natural human impulse to make all of these micro-adjustments has to be inhibited, because none of them helps. For example, you may temporarily improve the pain in your shoulders by throwing them back and lifting the front of your chest but you are hollowing and tensing the lower back by doing so. It doesn't improve the total pattern of your balance and postural alignment and it is just adding more tension to the system overall.

So you have to stop the natural human tendency to make things better by tensing your muscles and readjusting your body parts, but because you are a psycho-physical being it has to go even deeper than that. You have to stop even *wanting things to be different*. Do you see how subtle the Alexander Technique is? As long as there is still a desire, even a background wish, to make things better you are still in a state of tension because you are fighting what is happening at this point in time. You are in conflict with the reality of your experiences rather than accepting them and this causes mental and therefore some degree of physical tension as well. The directions will not flow if you are still holding at some level. To practise the Alexander Technique successfully what is actually needed is a special mode of thinking: non-judgemental awareness combined with letting go of any desire to change things. This is some of the subtlety contained in the meaning of those little words 'let' and 'allow'.

Personally when I am teaching new students about the Alexander Technique I prefer to be very explicit and up-front about my precise meaning and not leave things to chance. Which is why I have formulated an alternative form of directions, slightly different from Alexander's.

When you give directions you should always do so from a position of total self-acceptance. Even if there is an ache or pain behind that shoulder blade or in that knee, do not get into conflict with it and do not force it to change. That merely adds more tension (both mental and physical) to the situation and exacerbates it. Of course you do want it to change and to go away in the long term, but you have to be subtle about it. This strategy of change is really a form of paradoxical psychology. For example, if you are standing and wish to give directions with the long-term objective to release muscular tension and to lengthen your spine you could say something like:

> *"I am aware of this distance from the top of my head*
> *down to my ankles and heels.*
> *I am this tall, and I do not need to be any taller,*
> *and I do not need to be any shorter,*
> *I accept myself totally as I am,*
> *I do not have to change because everything is fine already."*

You see, the mind is a very tricky thing, but you have to be subtle and trick your mind. After all, why shouldn't you? Because your mind is tricking you all the time with all those subconscious assumptions and expectations that are running your life, just below the level of conscious awareness. So paradoxical psychology is essential when giving directions, and it isn't even a game any more because for that period of time whilst you are maintaining your directions, your thought projections, it actually has to be 100 per cent real and absolutely convincing for it to work, whilst you do not work, if you see what I mean.

Now maintain these thought projections for a period of time (at least 20-30 seconds, or better still, go into a timeless space); maintain that sense of ease and non-striving, and the muscular tension will suddenly release in its own time.

Now add directions to widen the back:

"I am this wide across the front of my chest,
along my collar bones and into my shoulder joints.
I am this wide across my back
from my spine across my shoulder blades and into
the shoulder joints,
to the left and to the right. I am this wide.
I don't need to be any wider or any narrower.
I accept myself totally as I am at this point in time.
I don't have to change anything because
I am perfect already."

Again, maintain these thought projections for at least 20-30 seconds, with a sense of calm awareness.

Finally add directions to free the jaw and neck muscles:

"I am aware that my jaw comes this far forwards to
the tip of my chin.
I am aware of this distance,
my jaw does not need to be any further forwards or
any more retracted.
I accept myself totally as I am at this point in time.
I don't have to change anything because everything
is fine already."

At the same time to free the neck:

"I am aware that my neck extends from my
shoulders up to the top joint where my head
balances on top of the spinal column.
My neck is the distance between my shoulders and my head.
My neck is this long and it doesn't need to be longer
or shorter.
It's fine just the way it is right now."

As you repeat these directions you may find that an extra
upthrust along the spine will be added to the flow of energy that you
already feel from the counter-thrust in your heels. You may also feel
(if you have already had Alexander lessons) that projecting these
directions has revived subconscious muscular memories of what it
felt like to have directions in your body during an Alexander lesson.
The important thing to realise is that you cannot force the
energy flow that comes as a result of giving directions. It comes in its
own time. That life energy is there all the time, and it will flow more
strongly as we mentally project the thought of these directions but

only when the conditions are right. There has to be an open channel for the energy to flow through. Just as water cannot flow through a hose pipe if there is even one tight bend that blocks the flow along the whole length of the pipe. There cannot be excessive tension in the muscles, or any sense of mental and emotional disharmony that would cause muscular tension somewhere in the system, because this muscular tension blocks the energy flow. Therefore, trying to force the experience that comes with the flow of directions is entirely counter-productive. Wanting it too much and getting impatient means that you are not accepting what is happening right now and therefore you are in a state of conflict and in a state of tension. This will block the flow of energy which is the very thing that you are trying to experience. It will never work that way, it just cannot be done.

If you haven't had lessons yet that is no reason not to try out the directions that I have described above. Maybe try projecting directions just down the right arm, from the shoulder to the elbow and onto the wrist and hand and fingertips, affirming, *"My arm is this long, from my shoulder to the tips of my fingers. It doesn't need to be longer or shorter, it's fine the way it is right now."* Maintain the projection of these directions for 30 seconds without wanting anything to be different and then compare your right arm with your left arm to see if there is any difference. Try the same experiment projecting directions along one leg only and then compare it to the other leg. Depending on your sensitivity and experience of subtle energy work in the body you might feel nothing, you might feel a subtle sense of lightness and a tingling sensation, or you might feel a really strong sense of flow, as if your leg is being lengthened and gently pulled out of your hip joint, or your arm out of the shoulder joint. If you feel something that's fine, and if you feel nothing that's also fine - but not a valid reason for stopping work with Alexander directions.

Actually Alexander was looking for a whole pattern of release throughout the body, where all the joints separate out and yet there is a feeling of overall integration through the free flow of connective directions. Crucial to this overall pattern of release is the way the head, neck and back align with each other, but there is a sense of balanced flow throughout the body. The full richness of this experience is hard to get without personal Alexander Technique lessons, but that is no excuse not to start practising the directions in the way that I have explained above.

Now after being in neutral for a small period of time you just forget about it all and carry on with your life. It's like driving a car, you put it into gear and away you go. But these directions have been impregnated into the muscular memory of your body and they are still working for you, even when your mind is occupied with something completely different.

Mental Calmness

The Alexander Technique does not work when you are tense, stressed and uptight. It is impossible because there is too much tension in the system. Which does not mean that you have to be lying on your back in a stress-free environment. Quite the contrary, there are many people who use the Alexander Technique when performing difficult and demanding tasks such as playing a musical instrument in front of an audience, or acting on stage, or giving a business presentation, or working in a stressful job. Mental attitude is more important than the situation you find yourself in; it is the determining cause of everything. Using the Alexander Technique gives you the self-confidence, the sense of inner self-respect, that allows you to perform your outer role convincingly. You have to learn how to be calmly active and actively calm, how to maintain your inner peace and calm under all conditions.

Now obviously there is a bit of a feedback loop here: you are practising your balance exercises, your breathing, and you are giving directions in order to feel calmer, and the calmer you are the smoother your mind works, with an increased attention span, and therefore you will be practising more successfully. That's clear. But I am also talking about any deep-seated mental or emotional conflicts, any stressful situations that are disturbing your peace and calmness and need resolving. (I shall be going into these in more detail in the chapter on psycho-physical rebalancing.) It is of little benefit using the Alexander Technique to continuously calm yourself down if there is some deeper issue that is continuously upsetting you. I remember one student of mine who would have her lesson and then go home and warn her husband, "Now, don't you go and say anything to upset me. I've just had a very expensive Alexander lesson and I don't want you ruining it all!" Actually it was no use blaming her husband. As long as she still had buttons to press she was bound to react when she got into those situations. She needed to understand the root cause of her reaction patterns, and change them. Which is not to absolve her husband from blame either, but merely to say that the way forward for her was to take responsibility for her own reaction patterns. You need constant vigilance if you wish to maintain your inner peace.

The precondition for maintaining your mental calmness is a different sort of thinking, a different level of consciousness. You actually need to be in a non-judgemental mode where you have the mental balance and clarity that can lead to a deep, calm state of inner awareness. A subtle key to this lies in the use of the eyes. If you observe people when they are being critical of someone else you will see how their eyes tend to harden and they will tense their eyeballs and the muscles around the eye sockets. It is a very hard, sceptical, critical look. Now, because you are a psycho-physical being, experiment with doing the opposite. Soften the focus of your gaze, soften your eyeballs, relax the muscles around your eye sockets. Let the light rays from the object or person you are looking at bounce off them and enter your eyeballs without any sense of grasping or strain. Keep the focus soft and keep the mind non-judgemental. This is not a state of blankness, this is actually a state of heightened awareness where you have gone beyond critical dualistic thinking. It's as if, looking at a person, you could think, "I accept this person exactly as they are, with all of their faults and virtues." It's as if, looking at an object, for example, a tree, you could think, "I accept this tree exactly as it is without thinking I like its shape or dislike its colour." Keep softening the gaze, keep relaxing the muscles around the eye socket, keep allowing the form and colour to register in a non-judgemental mind. Keep practising this psycho-physical exercise and notice if you feel different. You may well notice increased feelings of mental calmness, a greater sense of being fully present in the room and a sense of being fully identified with your sensory input in a non-judgemental way. This is called 'being in the flow'.

A key factor that works against this is being what Alexander called an 'end-gainer'. An 'end-gainer' is someone who is so stressed out with attaining their goal that they are unable to enjoy the present moment in time. Happiness is always at some far-off point in the future when some great ideal has been achieved. Of course, as this is a chronic habit, when they reach that point, there is a momentary sense of achievement before they must chase after the next goal - because happiness is always outside in material objects and acquisition which soon fades, and they do not know how to contact the happiness within. That sense of attunement comes from 'being in the flow', something that Alexander described as 'paying attention to the means whereby' (ie, the flow of directions) rather than being fixed on a future goal. Now look all around you in this society and what do you see? The pursuit of money, economic growth and mass production on a massive scale. So large that it is causing a breakdown of the planetary ecological system, and it is still not achieving that elusive goal of happiness. The first stage on the route to happiness is a balanced mental attitude and maintaining your inner peace and calmness.

PRIMARY CONTROL

Once these four preconditions - balance, breathing, directions, and mental calmness - are in place then you are in a position to experience the operation of 'primary control'. Primary control is very subtle; it is something that you allow to happen, but you can never force it. It is a state of consciousness, an energy flow more than an actual physical position, but we have to be clear about the precise location of the energy centre which is the heart of the phenomenon in order to work with it effectively. The source of primary control is in the medulla oblongata, which is that part of the brain where the brain stem tapers off into the spinal column. It is located just inside the atlanto-occipital joint where the head pivots on top of the spinal column.

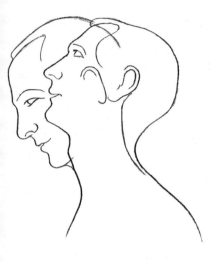

Figure 3

You can actually locate the atlanto-occipital joint more precisely by movement than you can by the study of anatomical diagrams. Just feel the little hollow at the back of your neck with your fingers and press into it as your head nods up and down as in Figure 3. That pivotal point is the atlanto-occipital joint. If you put a fingertip on either side of your head just below the ear lobes and continue nodding up and down slowly you will feel the axis of movement as the head nods on the atlanto-occipital joint. Notice how the movement comes from this top joint, lengthening the muscles at the back of the neck as you nod your head. It is not a movement that comes from C7, the seventh cervical vertebra, which is the one that sticks out prominently at the base of the neck. It is common to see people who, by mistake, have the habit of looking downwards by dropping the whole head and neck forwards from the base of the neck at C7. This drops the weight of the head (which is 10-12 lbs) too far forward and unbalances the whole body. If you have this habit you need to replace it immediately with the positive habit of looking down with a nodding movement from the top joint, as demonstrated in Figure 3. Actually, nature wants you to do this anyway, because the centre of gravity of the head is not directly over this joint, it is further forwards towards the front of the face. So the head will nod easily, it will nod forwards as you fall asleep on a bus or a train and all your muscles (including your neck muscles) relax. It will also nod slightly as you go over a bump, or in movement (such as walking) as your overall balance changes. This in turn affects the amount of tension you have in your neck muscles. As a result of this, and the large number of sensory nerve endings in the back of the neck, you have a feedback mechanism that helps you to orientate yourself in terms of bumps in the land and your movements in the space surrounding you. Also, due to the postural reflexes that are set off by this stretch along the back of the neck, there is a subtle reorganisation of muscles and posture throughout the body, thus the sense of stretch in the neck muscles also helps you to orientate yourself with regard to your inner bodily space. When trying to build computerised robots recently they found that they had to give them a neck with sensors built in, as well as eyes, or else the poor robot got badly disorientated as it moved through space. (Some design features just cannot be bettered and therefore can only be repeated!)

Now imagine what the consequences are if, due to poor posture or incorrect patterns of movement, these muscles at the back of your neck become permanently over-tensed. There is no flexibility there, no play, no contrast between tension and release, no subtle sensitivity that will enable you to coordinate your movements smoothly and orientate yourself correctly in terms of inner and outer space. You would be locked tight into the pseudo security of fixed patterns of movement with over-tensed muscles. That is why it is essential to have private Alexander Technique lessons. Through hands-on work during a lesson your Alexander Technique teacher should be able to give you the direct experience of what 'primary control' actually feels like - and it will be a revelation. The contrast with your earlier patterns of 'misuse' will be so great by comparison. There should be a sense of ease and lightness and a flow throughout the whole body; and when the neck muscles free up, the movement of the head on top of the spinal column should be so free that it appears to be almost weightless and effortless. It feels

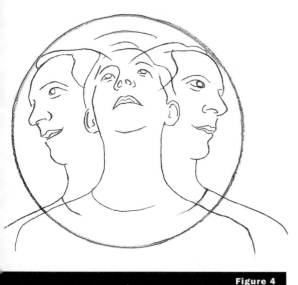

Figure 4

as if there is oil in the joint instead of rust and debris!

In the absence of a teacher try the head rotation exercise pictured in Figure 4 by yourself. Remember what was said earlier in this chapter about correct balance, breathing, directions and mental calmness. So stand or sit in a balanced position, take three slow, deep Alexander breaths, give directions along your total length and width and stay calmly focused.

Now just start to rotate your head slowly and consciously at the top joint using the minimum of muscle tension to do so. Do this a few times then reverse the direction. Speak to your neck muscles and ask them to use the minimum amount of tension to perform this rotation. Experiment with doing less. Speak to the muscles in the rest of your body and ask them to do nothing. Say, "You do not need to be involved in this movement, you are not involved, you can do nothing, it is only your neck muscles that need to work and they only need to do the minimum." Ask your neck muscles to do less and less, see what the minimum amount of tension really is. Keep alternating the direction of rotation.

Then stop and enjoy the sensation of having a freer neck. This is already the start of primary control. Through the physical exercise of rotating your head, in the manner described above, you can to some degree experience what it is like to have a freer neck and a more freely balanced head. However, this is only relative and when you go to a qualified and experienced Alexander Technique teacher for lessons you will be able to realise in progressively higher stages, what 'primary control' and the 'forward and up' really mean.

When the 'primary control' is open you can look through this opening as if it were a telescopic eye into the body and gain accurate information about the inner state of muscular tension or relaxation. What previously was a vague fog of murky physical sensations now becomes clarified and the precise pattern of muscular holding becomes clear. If you have precise information about what you are doing wrong then you are in a position to begin to release it with directions and to allow the right thing to happen, ie, a natural, balanced and aligned posture. Alexander always used to say, "Stop doing the wrong thing and the right thing will happen all by itself." *But first you have to know what the wrong thing is.* Primary control is an inner instrument of astonishing accuracy that allows you to know what the wrong thing is. For the Alexander Technique teacher primary control not only allows them to keep a check on their own pattern of use as they are working (ie, to see if any patterns of muscular tension are inadvertently creeping in) but also it allows the teacher to intuitively sense where the student is holding. This is felt as a parallel process of tension in the teacher's own body and it will release the instant the student releases. It works like magic and students often think that their teacher is telepathic, but actually it is just one of the many uses of primary control.

Primary control is also the most effective way to release tension throughout the body. Alexander makes it clear in his writings that the most effective way to deal with a specific area of tension is by first ensuring that the primary control is open. If, for example, you have a tension in your shoulders, you could deal with it by thinking a direction across the front of the chest along the collar bones, and also across the width of the back across the shoulder blades. Thinking directions whilst inhibiting at the same time would certainly bring about a certain degree of muscular release and a widening of the shoulders at some stage. However, it would be far more effective to first open up the primary control with directions and then from that centre of integration and release it is possible to direct a fresh flow of directions down the neck, across the width of the shoulders and then down the arms to the hands and the tips of the fingers. It is a really powerful flow of directions that you get from there and it works almost instantaneously to release over-tensed muscles and open up blockages. For seriously damaged or diseased body parts it naturally takes time for the body to heal, but the flow of directions, by creating muscular release, more space and easier circulation and respiration, is accelerating the body's natural healing process.

Alexander always used the little words 'allow' or 'let' at the start of his famous mantra:

> *"Allow the neck to be free,*
> *to let the head go forward and up*
> *to let the back lengthen and widen."*

I talked earlier about the importance of that little word 'let', and yet students tend to ignore it and skip onto 'the head go forward and up' and 'the back lengthen and widen'. This is natural because for years we have been taught that you get results by trying harder and we equate trying harder with over-tensed neck muscles and trying to force the end result. Now, if I ask one of my beginner students to 'let' their neck be free, almost inevitably they will start to tense their neck muscles; and if I say, 'Let the head go forward and up,' they will start to try and reposition their head in what they believe to be a forward and up position in space! This is an elementary mistake but one that often persists for a long time. So sometimes it is better just to say, "Don't pull your head back and down." Just don't do the wrong thing, that is all I ask of you at this stage. This simple order can be surprisingly effective.

Perhaps the easiest and most accurate way of freeing the neck (once you are familiar with the whole procedure of giving directions) is just to think:

> *"I am aware that my neck extends along my spine,*
> *from my shoulders up to the top joint where my head*
> *balances on top of the spinal column.*
> *My neck is the distance between my shoulders and my head.*
> *My neck is this long and it doesn't need to be longer*
> *or shorter.*
> *It's fine just the way it is right now."*

Maintain your awareness of these directions for at least 30 seconds without wanting anything to change. Stay in a balance position breathing calmly. At the same time you have to be giving directions to release the jaw muscles. These are some of the most powerful muscles in the body and if you try deliberately tensing your jaw muscles now you will see how that automatically tenses the back of your neck. As you release, the neck releases. So to release further you need to think a line along the jaw to the tip of the chin, and say to yourself:

> *"My jaw is this far forwards, it doesn't need to be further*
> *forwards or further retracted. I accept it, it is fine the way*
> *it is right now."*

Repeat this direction and hold the thought for at least 30 seconds, whilst you keep thinking directions to free the neck at the same time. Because the neck is lengthening whilst the jaw is releasing forwards, you may have created a tiny gap in the mid point, a bit more space, a sense of balanced release at the atlanto-occipital joint where the head balances on top of the spinal column. This is a very precise point and a very subtle opening takes place here. In the beginning it feels small and subtle, but later on it feels like a definite flow of energy and is much stronger. Once you have this sense of an opening you can think directions from there to anywhere in the body that is over-tensed or painful and blocked. That extra flow of energy will release and integrate your body.

You may perhaps now begin to experience the subtle sense of balance, the point of freedom that exists at the primary control. With practice and with the help of an experienced Alexander Technique teacher, that experience will undoubtedly grow stronger.

Once you have that sense of balance at the top joint, continue to give the rest of the directions to 'let the back lengthen and widen' to reinforce it because it is actually the whole of the head/neck/back relationship that constitutes the primary control. It is a continuous circle where each part strengthens and supports the next. Someone once asked Alexander which direction came first (ie, what is the most important causal element?) and he replied, "All together and one after another." Your awareness can remain with the whole cycle even though you are only dealing with one part specifically. Just as you can be juggling with several balls in the air at the same time even though you are only throwing one ball at a time. This is a very subtle skill but it comes with practice. It makes sense on an entirely practical level as well because the neck and shoulder muscles can only release properly when the spine is solidly grounded into the pelvis. Your sense of balance has to be rooted into something solid, and in this case it is the sense of the spine lengthening into the base of the pelvis and widening out into the width of the pelvis.

There is another subtle meaning to Alexander's directions which are rarely talked about and that is the expression 'to let the head go *forward and up*'. We have talked about the forward direction along the jaw, and the upward direction to the crown of the head. However, directions are not a position in space, they are more a movement of thought and energy. If we take the composite direction 'forward and up' it actually curves the energy forward from the primary control to the point between the eyebrows. This point corresponds to the 'third eye' in yoga and it has been known for thousands of years to be a centre of light, calmness, mental focus and spiritual thinking. So you can experiment with directing the energy along the spine from the base of the spine to just inside the hollow at the back of the neck. From there curve it forwards through the brain to the point between the eyebrows. Focus your awareness there and see what you feel.

Often there is a sensation of light, a feeling of great peace and calmness. The mind seems to work in a very clear, smooth and detached manner at this point. Very often you can find a reassuringly simple solution to a problem that you had been grappling with desperately just a moment ago. The solution had always been there; it is just that you had overlooked it in your panic and confusion. Now that the mind is working in a calm and focused manner you can see the obvious. Calmness is a quality that is often associated with the Alexander Technique, and this is the reason for it.

So through using directions and allowing the primary control to operate, it is possible to experience this calmness and to get in tune. You can be in the flow and take that unimpeded flow of energy, of calm awareness, into activity. It is not necessary to give directions the whole time; and, anyway, you have to get on and earn a living and focus on your work to be efficient. It would be impossible and undesirable to give directions all day long. But what you can do, and should do, is to use the little pauses in the day as they occur naturally, or just take a mini break of one or two minutes to practise some of the basic things that I have talked about in this chapter. Work with your balance, take three or four Alexander breaths. Give directions, open up the primary control, take your awareness forward and up to the point of calmness between the eyebrows. Allow that sense of peace to spread throughout all of your being, and then take that calmness into activity. As you carry on with your work and do whatever you have to do this day, whatever life is demanding of you, you can keep that sense of calmness in the background of your consciousness. Refuse to allow trivialities to upset you. Keep that mental focus and calmness going in the background, and you will find that you are keeping your directions flowing. It must be so because we are psycho-physical beings; no mental or emotional tensions means no physical blockages so the flow of directions can continue naturally. Take that calmness into activity and just go with it. If anything does happen to knock you badly off balance you know what you can do to rebalance yourself and get back in tune again.

In Figure 5 you can see an illustration of someone with primary control. You can notice that there is a head/neck/back alignment, the man seems balanced and calm and his eyes are looking forward and contacting the world. It would be impossible to convey more than that with a drawing or a photograph. Can you see what he is thinking, how he is breathing, what directions he is giving or what mental/emotional state he is in? Of course not, because that sort of information cannot be conveyed through the visual image to the inexperienced eye. But, you could sense it if you were in his presence. By the sense of touch, through the contact of hands-on work during the course of an Alexander

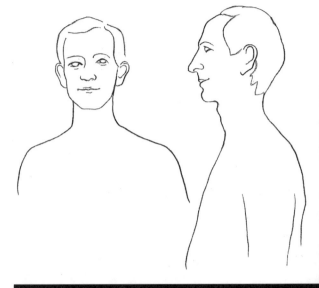

Figure 5

Technique lesson, the teacher is able to subtly convey the totality of the experience of primary control to the student - that is, information about the psycho-physical totality of being. We use words like 'presence' or 'personality' or 'aura' when we try to describe the whole being and the sense that they have something special. There is a famous story about A.R. Alexander (who was Alexander's brother and also an Alexander Technique teacher), sitting in a hotel lobby in Boston quietly smoking his pipe after a full day's teaching. Another guest in the hotel noticed something special about the whole quality of his being, so he went up to A.R. and said, "Sir, I don't know what it is that you have got, but I would sure like to have it." AR simply replied, "I bet you would," and then he got up and walked out of the lobby!

Chapter 5

AN ENERGY MODEL OF THE ALEXANDER TECHNIQUE

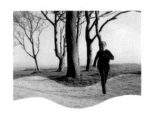

A lexander developed his Technique at the turn of the last century. It was the end of the Victorian era. He could not risk explaining his Technique in terms of energy or energy flow for fear of being misunderstood and ridiculed. He had developed his Technique in the comparative isolation of Australia -

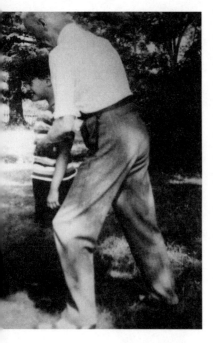

FM Alexander teaching a child the Alexander Technique

Alexander clearly maintains a free flow of energy throughout his body as he works on this young pupil. Notice how the upward thrust of energy along the spine and the freedom of the neck is clearly dependent on the whole back lengthening and widening and the stable base of the legs.

without the benefit of having read any books on Yoga or Tai Chi. He was a genius working on his own who had made a great discovery. He fitted his Technique into the prevailing scientific ethos of the time, which was predominantly scientific and mechanical. But he explained his Technique as a psycho-physical way of increasing poise and co-ordination by increased conscious control over the compulsive power of habitual reaction patterns through the use of the primary control. Indeed he called one of his books *Constructive Conscious Control of the Individual* to emphasise this point.

Many Alexander teachers talk of the 'flow', or the 'flow of energy' which results from directions. Patrick McDonald was one, and Misha Magidov is another. Any student who goes for a lesson with a good Alexander Technique teacher will certainly feel a sense of ease and lightness, a melting away of tension as the energy flow from directions releases and rebalances the whole body. The muscles are releasing and lengthening, the joints are opening, but there is also a tangible sense of life and energy, of tingling aliveness - like little pinpricks of light - as energy moves around the body in a marvellously subtle and intelligent manner. Indeed often the student will remark to their Alexander Technique teacher on how fine and exact their work has been and the teacher will deflect the praise with some modest and disparaging remark like, "Yes, that's what happens when you work with directions," because they know that at some fundamental level they are not doing the work. It is the flow of energy, directed by their thoughts that is doing the work; and this energy appears to be intelligent energy that flows to the place where it is needed and with just a little tweak here or a fine adjustment there it performs exactly the task that is needed, to perfection. Alexander Technique teachers in truth merely channel the energy to the required place; because whilst they know through their observations that the back in general needs lengthening or the shoulders need widening, etc, they will give directions for this, but the precise mechanics of how that is achieved is left to the flow of life energy which performs its task to perfection. Nothing is overdone and nothing is left undone, and like the sweet progression of a Mozart sonata, the work flows onwards towards a conclusion of perfect balance and harmony.

How can we explain what happens during the course of an Alexander lesson? There are several different theoretical models that can explain the experience of the Alexander Technique. The traditional model explains the Technique in terms of the skeleton, muscles, the hard-wired nervous system and mental 'orders' from the brain to the various body parts (which is what 'directions' are understood to be). The new energy model of the Alexander Technique proposes something fundamentally different. It proposes that we are living in a sea of cosmic energy, that surrounds us and permeates us, that this is the sustaining force behind all life forms and the energy blueprint for all growth and expansion. There is both a universal sea of energy and our own individual reservoir of life energy that is unique to each person. While we are alive our bodies are operating on this individual reservoir of life energy and we can top up our energy through subsidiary sources such as food, water, air and sunshine. When we are dead the life force has gone and nothing will restore life to the body. However, if you learn the Alexander Technique or any other form of *pranayama* technique (literally, 'control of life force' technique) then you are able to replenish your individual reserves of life energy by tapping into the infinite ocean of life energy that surrounds us. Alexander's discovery of the 'primary control' (at the medulla oblongata where the brain stem tapers off into the spinal column) is the discovery of how to open the main gate through which this energy can flow into the body. This life energy is not ours to own and control like we can own money or possessions, but we can learn to cooperate and work with it. It is an energy flow that can be directed by our thoughts. But the fact that most people cannot see it doesn't mean that it isn't there; and even if you cannot see it, it doesn't mean that you cannot *feel* it and learn to work with it.

You *can feel* the exquisite flow of directions in your own body during the course of an Alexander session, and *you can feel* the warm, soothing flow of directions that drop like a flow of golden honey from the hands and fingers of an experienced Alexander teacher. Some people may not be sensitive enough to be aware of it, but enough (a significant majority) are aware of what is happening, and this combined with the intensity of the experience is enough to convince me that awareness of energy flow is not a subjective experience. You can perform a simple experiment for yourself now to see if you can sense your life force or not.

1) Relax the shoulders and arms.

2) Cup your hands in front of you as if you are holding a ball. Find the distance that feels right for you. Starting from far away slowly move the hands closer together until at a certain point you may feel that the air thickens up into a sponge-like feeling that slightly pushes the hands away from each other.

3) Stay there for a while allowing the energy charge to build up until it feels like you have a warm, round ball of energy between your hands.

4) Play with it; what do you want to do with it?

5) Experiment with tensing and then releasing your shoulders, elbows or wrists; how does this affect the ball of energy between your hands?

From my experience of teaching Alexander Technique classes about 70 per cent of students are able to sense this ball of energy between the hands.

Alexander suggested another form of experiment to show the power of directions.

He instructed his readers to simply lay out both hands flat on a table whilst sending directions down to the tip of each index finger but ignoring the other fingers and thumbs. He suggested that the best way to do this was by thinking of a potential movement of the index fingers whilst refusing to make any movement or to tense the muscles at all. If you try this experiment for a minute or two the index fingers begin to feel very alive and warm and tingling. The other fingers and thumbs appear almost asleep by comparison!

Now how can we explain that feeling of aliveness and energy that comes from directions? You could just say that it is the result of a relaxed muscle tone and increased blood supply, and stick to a very mechanical model of the Alexander Technique. If you are happy with that model and your view of the world does not include the concept of 'life energy' flow then that is fine and the Alexander Technique as it stands will still continue to work for you. Directions, just like gravity, will continue to work whatever your belief system might be. However, I believe that there is more to it than that.

There is so much of the Alexander Technique that could obviously be explained by energy flow. Many of the thoughts and images used are ways of building up an energy charge and then being able to channel that energy in a useful direction. Many teachers speak of *"keeping the back back"* and Patrick McDonald would talk of sending directions "up along the spine". I often encourage my clients to walk backwards around the room in order to experience what *keeping the back back* feels like and I will then continue working on them with directions in order to heighten the experience. You can allow the energy charge to build up in the back in this way. Some Alexander Technique teachers, I think Misha Magidov was the first, use the powerful image of the back being like a tank full of water (water = energy), with the arms joined like pipes at the shoulders (but without tension anywhere), so as to allow a free flow of 'water' through to the hands and fingertips and into the body of the client. We can never control or force the flow of energy - we can only allow it to happen. So we just calmly keep on giving directions without expecting any results. Now, however, comes the subtle bit. When things do start happening, as both teacher and pupil can begin to feel the muscles releasing and the body getting deliciously soft, warm and tingling with aliveness, the tendency is for the ego to step in and to start getting excited and wanting to take credit for the whole thing. This is a fundamental error because any mental excitation immediately causes tension and blocks the whole flow. The whole story just stops there. The experienced teacher however is able to stay even-minded and detached from the excitation of his ego and just calmly keep on sending directions without getting involved in any way, taking the client deeper and deeper and allowing the whole process to reach a greater level of power and intensity. The process stays open-ended and both the teacher and the client are pleasantly surprised by the new territory that has been visited. Indeed, the client often comments, "I don't think that I have ever managed to release that so much in my life before."

If you look at Kirlian photographs of the hands of an Alexander teacher or a healer when their mind is preoccupied with some trivial problem, compared with when they are calmly focused on giving directions or healing work, the difference is phenomenal. Kirlian photography shows the electromagnetic force field surrounding the body; and while it does not show the actual life force it shows how our thoughts have affected the life force which in turn clearly influences the electromagnetic force field surrounding the body. Something is clearly happening on an energetic level when you give directions, not only within your body but also in the space surrounding your body.

Now two fundamental characteristics of this life energy are: a) that it is intelligent, and b) that it responds to our thoughts. This then becomes the fundamental explanatory principle of the Alexander Technique. In the energy model of the Technique 'directions' = thought projections = energy flow. In other words *through our thoughts we can direct the energy flow* within our bodies, and within the bodies of our clients. This is what gives the Alexander Technique its power and its subtlety. On the surface nothing much is happening during the course of a lesson. It would certainly make a very boring film! But underneath there is so much going on in terms of muscular releases, subtle energy flows and the opening and integration of different parts of the body.

The other fascinating thing about the Alexander Technique is that the Alexander teacher is in tune with what is happening inside the body of the pupil. The teacher can be working on the head and neck of the pupil and say, "You have just released your left knee," or, "You have just dropped your shoulders," or, "You have just grounded yourself and connected with your legs and feet." At first the pupil thinks that the teacher has very good powers of observation, and this may be the case, but then he will realise that sometimes the teacher is just too far away to have noticed such small physical changes, and besides it is also happening instantaneously, because the teacher is often *telling him about changes at the very instant that they are occurring in his body.* Something is happening that needs closer examination here. I believe that it is due to the energetic link that occurs with hands-on treatment. It is the equivalent to the counter-transference in psychotherapy. By coming into close contact with the pupil, and especially once he places his hands anywhere on his pupil, the Alexander teacher knows exactly where his pupil is holding muscular tension, *because he feels it in his own body.* How can we adequately explain this phenomenon? Only through the concept of a life energy field that surrounds and penetrates each living person. This is like an energy blueprint that shows the physical, mental and emotional habit patterns of that individual. The Alexander teacher is like a blank slate, trained to be mentally calm and physically released, so that when these disturbing patterns suddenly appear he knows immediately, "This is not me, this is my pupil," and he now has valuable information to work with during the course of the session. The teacher is trained to carry on giving directions in his own body to release that particular tension pattern. The

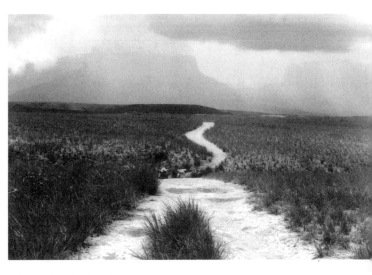

Mountains in the Mist

Great landscapes have the capacity to awaken in us a sense of awe and wonder. 'The nameless is the beginning of Heaven and Earth.'

instant that body part releases he knows that it has also released in the body of his pupil and he can comment on it and make it part of the learning of that session. This intuitive sense of knowing cannot be explained by physical sensations alone because it is too precise and works even at a distance. This attunement can only be explained by an energetic connection transmitted through life energy. If you have the capacity to stay mentally calm and to pay attention to this subtle intuitive knowledge then this sense can be trained and it becomes a source of vitally important information.

What is this energy? Where does it come from? Where does it flow to and what is its purpose? Who can say? Certainly not with words because these are questions about the big fundamental issues of life. With words we can never capture the essence of a thing nor the reality of an experience. Words are only symbols that point the way and can never become the thing itself. The Tao Te Ching makes this point beautifully.

"The Tao that can be told is not the eternal Tao.
The name that can be named is not the eternal name.
The nameless is the beginning of heaven and earth.
The named is the mother of ten thousand things.
Ever desireless, one can see the mystery.
Ever desiring, one can see the manifestations.
These two spring from the same source but differ in name;
this appears as darkness.
Darkness within darkness.
The gate to all mystery."

(Tao Te Ching, poem 1)

The advice from the Tao Te Ching is to learn to go with the flow, rather than name and classify it. Merge yourself into it, but do not desire to control it or ask too many questions. Remain merged in the flow without desires, in a state of creative indifference, and all will be revealed in time!

The ancient Chinese sages found it just as difficult to write about the Tao as I do to write about the ultimate meaning of the flow of life energy that is experienced during the course of an Alexander lesson. Why? Because this energy is life force, it represents the primordial unity of life, which is God, or the Tao, or the Cosmos or whatever limiting and inadequate name you want to give to the Creator, the beginning and end of all creation, the sustainer and the destroyer of universes, who is unknowable by the purely intellectual mind. The only way we can begin to experience God is through an intuitive energy approach. That is why an Alexander Technique lesson can be such a profoundly satisfying experience, because we have tasted something of God. By learning to control and direct the life force, turning the flow inwards so that it is concentrated within the spine, we find the interior, esoteric way to God through higher intuitive experiences. A good introduction is to have a lesson with an experienced Alexander Technique teacher who can give you the direct experience of a 'pranayama' technique, what it is like to have the energy flowing up and down the spine - don't expect too much and don't discount the experience as being too subtle. It is only the beginning of a long journey.

We can observe the flow of life force in nature. It is the creative and sustaining force behind all life forms, all growth and expansion. Who can fully explain the miracle of a seed and the way it grows into a plant? There is an intelligent energy that provides a blueprint for the growth and development of all living forms from the highest to the lowest. Nature becomes like an open book to read when we understand this secret and begin to observe its operation. We can contact the power of this life force in plants, animals and beautiful landscapes. Even in the desert, a desert landscape is not empty but is buzzing with life force. Look what happens when it rains and the vital element of water is added, the desert just explodes into life for a short period of lush beauty and growth. You can feel that potential, because the life force is there at all times, even in the dry periods. We think that man lives by food and by oxygen alone but it is not true. Take a dead man and stuff his stomach full of food and blow his lungs up with fresh oxygen but he will not come back to life. What is missing is the life force that has left that form. The Bible says, "Man shall not live by bread alone but by every word that proceedeth from the mouth of God" (Matthew 4: 4). "The mouth of God" is a reference to the medulla oblongata, where the brain stem tapers off into the spinal column. This is exactly the point that

Alexander called the 'primary control' and he said it needed to be open to allow a free flow of directions (= life energy) throughout the body. If you are alive each person has their own individual reservoir of life force within the body, which is replenished indirectly by food, water, oxygen and sunshine, but by learning esoteric Yoga techniques, or by learning about the 'primary control' in the Alexander Technique you can replenish your individual supply of life force from the infinite ocean of energy that surrounds you. This is certainly the most direct way of increasing your health and vitality levels!

To my mind this energy can only satisfactorily be described as 'life energy' or 'life force'. It is described in all the ancient Taoist texts and worked with in Acupuncture and Tai Chi. In China they called it 'Chi' or life energy. From the serene and surprisingly modern-looking sculptures that have survived from ancient Egypt (see picture) it is obvious that they knew how to sit and meditate and the wonderful openness of the posture shows that they knew how to give directions and open up the full length and width of the torso. Because the high priests and pharaohs knew how to leave the body during meditation and to return to it after travel in the astral spheres, the ordinary Egyptians could never be sure if such a person was really dead or might wish to return to the body at some future date. The practice of mummification was to allow the person's 'Ka', or life energy, to return into the mummified body if needed and to bring the body back to life to provide a home for the 'Ka' and the spirit self, if they were not really

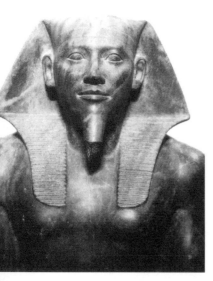

Pharaoh Kafre

The power and serenity of the Pharaohs who were the spiritual, political and military leaders of their societies, is shown in this sculpture of Kafre, builder of the second great pyramid. His calm confidence is revealed in the wonderful openness of his shoulders.

dead after all. In the Hindu tradition they called it 'Prana', or life force, and it is an essential part of Yoga and all meditation forms to learn to control this energy flow. There are well-documented reports of Hindu sages being buried alive for weeks or even months in a state of suspended animation and then calmly walking away once they had been dug up again and the life energy had re-entered the body.

There can be no true meditation without 'Pranayama' or life force control. In all the ancient civilisations where higher spiritual knowledge was retained they knew how to work with this energy as a form of healing, and how to direct the energy up along the spine to awaken the chakras and attain a higher level of consciousness. (See Chapter 10 on the spiritual dimension of the Alexander Technique.) The Alexander Technique, in one sense, is a reawakening of this ancient knowledge of how to direct life energy into a body part when it needs healing, or through the innermost spinal channel (the Susumna) if we wish to awaken the centres of higher knowledge.

This life energy is also the power that heals; and all great healers have known how to channel and direct this energy. In the New Testament there are many vivid accounts of Christ's work as a healer. Through the healing power of touch the greatest amount of life force is transferred. Jesus was in a crowd once when a woman came up and touched him from behind because she wanted healing. Jesus turned around and said, "Who has touched me for I feel virtue has gone out of me?" By *'virtue'* he meant the life force within him that had flowed into the woman and had healed her. He felt the loss and she felt the gain and was healed. His loss was only temporary, however, because he had the technique of how to replenish himself from the infinite source.

The Martial Arts also work with Chi energy. The Aikido master stays perfectly calm and centred as he uses the life force to turn his opponent's energy against him and to throw him. The Karate expert can chop a brick or a thick piece of wood with his hand but it isn't the physical blow that breaks it, it is the power of the 'Chi' energy extending beyond the hand that breaks the block *before the hand hits it.* Another simple experiment from the Martial Arts that you can perform with a partner is to stretch out an arm in front of you with the palms upwards and allow your partner to gauge your strength as he tries to bend it upwards from the elbow. He can push up with one hand under your hand and the other one on the inside of the arm at your elbow joint, whilst you resist using physical strength alone. Now do the same thing, except first think 'directions' along the length of the arm out to the tips of the fingers until you feel calmly connected. Now keeping that connection flowing through to the fingertips and keeping the shoulders relaxed resist, your partner's attempts to bend your arm. If you are doing this right he will be totally unable to bend your arm at all, because life force is stronger than physical strength every time.

An interesting group experiment that I have conducted with my dance and drama students is the 'levitation' experiment where one volunteer is asked to lie out flat on a table and a group of 10 or 12 students surrounds that person. The object of the exercise is for the group to lift the person lying horizontally on the table easily and lightly just using the tips of their fingers if possible. As a preparation the group will visualise the person as being light as a feather and the lifting to be easy, flowing and effortless. The whole group rubs their hands for a minute to stimulate the flow of life energy to the fingertips. Then they all hold hands in a circle around the figure on the table to create a group energy field and to get the energy flowing through the shoulders and the arms. At the right point in time, when the breath has calmed down sufficiently and the mind is clear and focused, the whole group steps forward (preferably in a lunge position with one foot stepping forwards and the back foot opening out slightly) and, bending easily at the knees and the hips, they slide their fingers under the body of the person on the table and lift them up high in one smooth motion. If this has all been done correctly there is an immediate group sensation of, "This is so easy, I can't believe how light this person is!" The danger is that some people in the group will start giggling or exclaiming loudly at this point, but if you can keep your mental focus and not get excited the life energy will continue flowing smoothly and you can easily hold the person up there for a period of time before gently lowering them back to the table again. The most amazing thing, however, is the experience of the person on the table. They will often report a feeling of lightness, like being lifted on a wave of energy and suspended in mid air before gently parachuting back down to the ground again.

The concept of life energy is universal. Its existence has been part of the higher knowledge of all ancient civilisations. Alexander merely rediscovered something that has been known about for a long, long time. As our spiritual and scientific knowledge increases Alexander's discovery will be seen in its true perspective: as a rediscovery of how to work with the energy body that interpenetrates and surrounds the physical human body. We can direct this energy with the power of our thoughts and it is more powerful than merely muscular strength. However, the state of mind of the practitioner is crucial; you cannot direct this energy flow in an agitated or disturbed state of mind. The waves of mental and emotional excitation have to calm down to a state of pure awareness. Personal ego motivations have to be overcome *so that the practitioner is totally unconcerned about the outcome.* A state of calm attunement and pure awareness is needed. Time disappears, the consciousness is lifted beyond the dualities of good or bad, success or failure. The outcome of the session is totally unimportant because you are now existing in a deepened awareness of the eternal NOW. Everything just is, and it is perfect already in its essence (even though sometimes the surface conditions may not appear to be optimal). Underlying it all flows a river of peace and harmony. Tune in with *the flow* by whatever means you can, work with it and you will experience the truth, that 'all is well and all shall be well'.

UNDERSTANDING ALEXANDER'S TERMINOLOGY

The Alexander Technique is certainly one of the oldest and most beautiful methods of working with the whole psycho-physical organism of the human being. Alexander brought his technique to this country in 1904, and as many other holistic therapies have developed since then (some of them undoubtedly influenced by Alexander's work, such as the Feldenkreis Method), the Alexander world has tended to withdraw into insularity, emphasising the uniqueness of its methodology and the purity of its results rather than attempting to build bridges and explore areas of common understanding. Indeed, there is an ongoing debate in the Alexander community as to whether the Alexander Technique is to be classified along with other alternative and complementary health treatments, or whether it is a system of re-education that should be placed in the educational sphere. Opinion is divided, but my view (which is apparently shared by publishers, bookshops and the general public) is that the Alexander Technique should be firmly placed in the Alternative Health category, amongst other body/mind therapies, and should not be marginalised by being placed in the educational sphere.

Whilst I firmly believe that the Alexander Technique has therapeutic benefits and that we are working with the life force, like all the other alternative therapies, I think it is important to continue with the tradition of calling ourselves 'teachers' in the sense that we are teaching people a methodology, a technique and a process of working, which we hope a person will be able to go away with to practise and use on their own. So in that sense it is correct to call an Alexander Technique practitioner a 'teacher' (which is also a term of respect), rather than a 'therapist'.

The main problem with understanding Alexander's terminology is that some of the language of the Technique, as originally formulated by Alexander in his books, has become very dated and misleading. One of the key obstacles is that the use of language can develop over time, and particular words can change their meaning due to frequent usage in a particular context. The most obvious example is in the way the word 'inhibition' has changed its meaning since the Freudians started using it in the context of 'inhibiting' emotional expression or sexuality, and it has acquired a negative connotation.

In addition we have the problem that words can never give you the experience of the thing they describe; they can only stand as a symbol of the actual experience. This makes them prone to misinterpretation and inaccuracies. How can I explain to someone what an apple tastes like who has never tasted an apple? I can get close, but we will never really be talking the same language until we have had the same experience. In this sense, all words, all books about the Alexander Technique, are misleading and useless compared to having a course of Alexander Technique lessons with a qualified and experienced teacher, who can give you direct experience.

Having said that, there are obviously people who don't have the time for lessons and just want to read a good introductory text; or, having had lessons with a teacher, they may wish to put their experience into a clear theoretical framework. I feel that one of the major obstacles to increased public understanding of the Technique today lies in Alexander's naturally dated use of language and obscure explanations of the core concepts. This can prevent people from linking up to the validity of their own inner experiences, or from building bridges to other alternative therapies or spiritual techniques that they may have practised. So many gems of wisdom are hidden in Alexander's rather ponderous and long-winded Victorian style of writing that I feel it is important to winnow out the truth and explain it in simple, modern language, so that the modern reader can clearly understand it - and not only understand it but put it into practice. So in this chapter I am writing an updated description of the core concepts of the Alexander Technique and proposing a few new terms. Of course it could be that some people will find Alexander's original terminology preferable and in that case they should carry on using it. I will continue using the original terms in this book, but I will also be proposing and using some new terminology in the hope that this will lead to a deeper understanding of the core concepts.

'Giving Directions': Directions are really just *thought projections,* that is, lines of thought that are maintained steadily in awareness for a period of time. Thought is energy because where the thoughts go the energy follows, so the life energy within the body is effectively being guided by thoughts to different areas of the body to relax muscles, improve the posture and restore general ease of functioning. A typical 'direction' would be from the base of the spine to the crown of the head to *allow* the back to lengthen, and from the sternum across the chest into the shoulder joints to *allow* the front of the chest to widen. I am going to use both terms interchangeably. Alexander's original term of 'directions' is not bad because it does imply that you can direct the energy with your thoughts. It also has a secondary meaning of directions as in 'pointing to', so we are pointing to the primary directions of up and down, left and right, forwards and backwards.

'Inhibition': This is not to be confused with the Freudian term and all its connotations of sexual and emotional repression. Inhibition basically means to stay perfectly relaxed physically and not to react in your habitual mode. On one level it means just saying "No" and refusing to react, but it also means maintaining a lively level of interest and awareness at the same time as you are saying no. So it actually means a lot more than the words 'inhibition' or 'saying No' would imply, and I would prefer the term *creative indifference.* Alexander always emphasised that directions should be combined with inhibition; or in my proposed new terminology that 'thought projections' should always be combined with a mental state of 'creative indifference'. The meaning immediately becomes clearer, does it not? If we are to mentally project energy, the thoughts must be held steady and clear. There must be no tension and no negativity. To take a specific example, if my back muscles are tensed or damaged and I wish to release and lengthen my back I would project the thought, "I am this tall from the base of the spine at the coccyx right up to the crown of the head." For this thought to work effectively I would need all the muscles to remain perfectly relaxed, and to remain mentally and emotionally relaxed, refraining from blaming my back muscles for being tense and painful. Therefore I would combine it with the thought, "I am this tall and I do not want to be taller or shorter. I do not have to change anything because it is perfect already." With this thought process there is no blame, no conflict and no added tension. I am remaining in awareness, in a state of creative indifference, without striving. As I do so, suddenly when I least expect it, as if from nowhere, there is a release (that is felt simultaneously by both the pupil and the Alexander teacher) and the back releases and lengthens. This is termed 'non-doing'. Why? Because there has been no physical doing or manipulation by anyone; the energy flow, stimulated by thought projection, has done the work. One word of warning, any impatience or desire to check and see if the thought projections really are working or not is counter-productive because it leads to doubt and tension. You really do have to remain 100 per cent in a state of inner creative indifference.

'End-Gaining': Alexander's term is aptly descriptive. This refers to that part in us which fixes its sight on a goal and strives towards it no matter what the cost might be. Alexander's observations of his pupils led him to the conclusion that most of the mental and muscular holding that was occurring was due to the habit of being so intent on reaching some particular goal in the future that the present could not be adequately enjoyed at all. This led him to formulate the next concept.

Paying attention to **The Means Whereby** I would call *being in the flow* or paying attention to *the creative process.* As I sit here typing this chapter on my word processor I can either: think, "I can't wait until this article is finished; I'll be so happy and then I can rest or go for a walk in the sunshine" thus deferring my happiness until some future point; or, I can sit here staying relaxed and balanced and enjoying the creative process as it occurs, that inner buoyant feeling, feeling connections being made, watching the odd creative thought bubbling up and bursting onto the surface of my consciousness, feeling 'in tune', as if my thoughts are being directed almost without my conscious effort. I am feeling alive and happy RIGHT NOW and I'm enjoying what I'm doing. As an Alexander Technique teacher I know that I am a psycho-physical being and that I cannot actually get into this state unless I have both the correct mental attitude and am physically poised and relaxed.

'Faulty Sensory Appreciation': is an accurate descriptive term that refers to Alexander's brilliant insight that most people suffer from inaccurate sensory awareness. Because a particular posture or muscular tension pattern is habitual, after a time it is accepted as 'normal' and it is no longer noticed by the conscious mind. This however does not make it right or normal; it is just that the mind has filtered out any messages from the sensory nerve endings to the contrary. Even though it is wrong, it feels right; and conversely what is right will feel wrong. Thus it is that often after an Alexander Technique teacher has corrected a client's balance and postural alignment the client will complain about feeling out of balance and 'wrong', and only when taken to view themselves in a mirror will they see for the first time that they are in fact in their correct alignment.

'Primary Control': I would prefer the term *free flow of life energy*. When there is a perfect balance of the head on top of the spinal column, extra life energy can flow in through the medulla oblongata, which is the bottom part of the brain where it tapers off into the spinal column. When all the prerequisites have been met: deep, calm abdominal breathing, perfect balance throughout the whole line of the body, calmness, awareness, feeling incredibly centred and grounded in the pelvis and legs - then the Alexander Technique teacher is able to use directions to open up the *free flow of life energy* throughout the body. There is a point of freedom at the fulcrum, or balance point, and this is also a point of release. Through this point of freedom we can allow an inflow of extra life energy into the body, through the medulla oblongata. Life force can flow through into the brain, into the spine and all the body parts. Through the subtle opening of the medulla at this point life energy can then be directed to flow into any part of the body that needs healing or releasing. The medulla incidentally is the only part of the body that cannot be operated on: if a surgeon were to accidentally cut it with a scalpel the patient would die immediately.

I hope that this explanation of Alexander's terminology will be of some benefit to readers, and that the proposed changes will help to make the Alexander Technique more accessible and understandable to a wider range of people. The important thing is that you should use whatever terms resonate and make the most sense for you personally.

Chapter 6

LET YOUR LIFE FLOW - INTO MOVEMENT

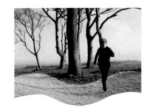

When you first start trying to integrate the Alexander Technique into your daily life there may be a tendency to stiffen the spine and tense the muscles as you try to position your head and neck and shoulders in a certain way or to hold a certain alignment of the spine. This may be done because you have seen photographs of models in Alexander Technique books with superb poise and alignment demonstrating how to apply the Technique in different situations, and you naturally want to imitate them. Or perhaps you have been taught something in your Alexander Technique lesson and you are trying to reproduce the experience by holding yourself in a certain position. Any held position, especially when it is being done for the supposedly laudable motive of trying to be a 'good student' and please your teacher, is total anathema to the principles of the Alexander Technique. A held position means that your muscles are tensed and there can be no energy flow, no flow of directions through over-tensed muscles. You have the shell but not the essence of the Technique. It cannot work that way because there is no living flow to carry the posture from within. That is why a photograph is so dangerous, because it is only one snapshot taken during a whole flow of movement. Most importantly it cannot show what the person is thinking or what their state of consciousness is.

Illustrations have been deliberately chosen for this section rather than photographs because they are softer and give more of the feel of a movement rather than a photographically exact image to be imitated. Remember, no one has perfect posture, no one is exactly symmetrical. You are not here to achieve perfection in the outer form, but rather in the inner form. I will be showing you certain sequences of movement that I would like you to practise in your daily life. These are 'exercises' in the sense that they need daily repetition, but not exercises in the way that people go to the gym to exercise. They are exercises in the sense of a bodily, mental and spiritual training, a discipline, a path on the way to inner perfection. If we look at the Oxford Dictionary definition of the word exercise it comes from a Latin root *exercitium* which means both to *restrain* and *keep at work*. I use the word in this sense. You need to restrain the ego with its desire to get it right and to seek praise and acknowledgement from others, whilst you keep on working according to the principles that have been explained to you.

Ultimately what you are seeking is a state of non-doing in activity - a movement that does itself through pure energy flow, freed from the bondage of the fearful and constricting ego. As long as there is still a flicker of the thought - Am I getting it right? Will my teacher praise or blame me? Will my friends admire me or despise me? - you are still in ego mode and bound to fail because of unnecessary mental and muscular tension in the system. The more your consciousness can detach itself from the ego with all its plans for greatness and its fear of failure, promising happiness at the end of the tortured trail (which is a lie!), the more you will know what I mean.

The purpose of *exercitium* is gradually, through practice and self-observation, to perform these movements with less and less muscular tension, to move towards a state of pure awareness of the moment, enjoying the sense of flow in these movements for their own sake, from a non-judgemental standpoint. The paradox is, of course, that all the happiness we are seeking is within us already, at this present moment in time, rather than at some illusory point in the future when we have achieved all our goals and are finally worthy of praise. So stick to the principles and 'allow' things to happen rather than try to get it right!

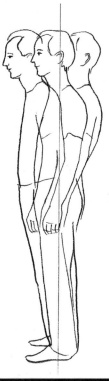

Figure 6

The first principle is the principle of balance. One of the basic ideas of the Alexander Technique is how to release into balance rather than to hold yourself rigid in a preconceived idea of what your correct postural alignment should be. Look at Figure 6 and notice how the optimal line of balance should pass through the crown of the head, the atlanto-occipital joint where the head balances on top of the spine, through the centre of gravity in the abdomen and down through the ankles and heels and into the ground. Balance is a living thing, you need to play with it and discover every day, either standing or sitting, where your balance line is today.

A pregnant woman will find that her postural alignment needs to change every day as her baby grows out to the front. Your posture and therefore your optimal line of balance is changing every day as well. You may not realise where your optimal line of balance is because you are holding yourself in a habitual way, which feels right but is wrong. Use a mirror, sway backwards and forwards, play with different positions until you really do find the place where you can feel the counter-thrust from the ankles and heels. It is that energy that should be carrying your posture, not muscular tension.

It is the same when sitting at your desk and writing on a computer keyboard. Take time every now and then (say every hour) to just sway backwards and forwards from the hip joints until you come to an optimal balance point where the crown of your head is balanced over your sitting bones at the bottom of the pelvis. So the calmness and solidity of the pelvis support a strong spine with the head balanced on top. Then *keep your back back* by imagining a big cushion of air behind your whole back, allowing you to release all of your back muscles as if you were lying on the ground. Give directions along the length of the spine, from the crown of the head to the bottom of the pelvis:

> *"I am aware of this distance from the top of my head*
> *down to my ankles and heels.*
> *I am this tall, and I do not need to be any taller,*
> *and I do not need to be any shorter,*
> *I accept myself totally as I am,*
> *I do not have to change because everything is fine already."*

and across the width of the shoulders:

> *"I am this wide across the front of my chest,*
> *along my collar bones and into my shoulder joints.*
> *I am this wide across my back*
> *from my spine across my shoulder blades and into*
> *the shoulder joints,*
> *to the left and to the right. I am this wide.*
> *I don't need to be any wider or any narrower.*
> *I accept myself totally as I am at this point in time.*
> *I don't have to change anything because*
> *I am perfect already."*

Allow three deep Alexander breaths *to flow* and release your stomach muscles. Remember, the important point in Alexander breathing is that the lungs need to be emptied completely during exhalation. If there is any effort used, and sometimes there does need to be a bit of effort at the start of a breathing exercise, the effort should go into ensuring that all the air is fully expelled from the lungs, especially the bottom lobes. Then you have to let go and allow the air to flow in all by itself, without any sense of will-power or muscular effort being used. The point is that if all the air has been fully expelled as the ribcage contracts and the diaphragm relaxes and returns to its top position then a partial vacuum has been created in the lungs and atmospheric pressure outside will push the air back into the lungs, through the nose or mouth, in order to equalise the pressure outside and inside the ribcage. Once you have breathed out fully, atmospheric pressure will do its stuff and refill your lungs with air. You do not have to do anything to help.

Give directions to free up the primary control:

> *"I am aware that my neck extends along my spine,*
> *from my shoulders up to the top joint where my head*
> *balances on top of the spinal column.*
> *My neck is the distance between my shoulders and my head.*
> *My neck is this long and it doesn't need to be longer*
> *or shorter.*
> *It's fine just the way it is right now."*

and also to release the jaw:

> *"My jaw is this far forwards,*
> *it doesn't need to be further forwards*
> *or further retracted.*
> *I accept it, it is fine the way it is right now."*

Look at the way the man is sitting in Figure 7, you can sense that he has come to a point of balanced equilibrium, not just in terms of physical alignment but also in terms of his inner mental and emotional processes. Sitting serenely like this takes practice. There is no quick fix and instant gratification for the ego because we are actually battling to get rid of the ego and reach a state of calm acceptance and pure awareness. After a minute or two's practice swing forward very slightly from the hip joint, drop the chin gently, as if nodding your head, so that you can look down at your paperwork, the computer screen or keyboard, and carry on with your writing. You will find that whatever job you are working at will go more smoothly because the emotions are calm and the mind is clear and focused.

Now look at the exercise in Figure 8. The legs are spread wider than a shoulder's width apart and the man is standing in his optimal balance line, with his *back back* and his weight travelling down through his ankles and heels. Get into this alignment, feel that you are grounded and balanced. Give

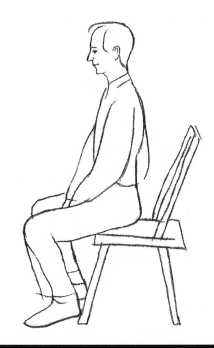

Figure 7

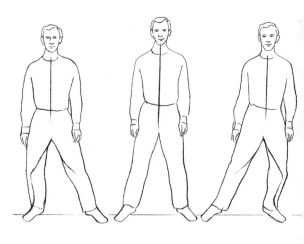

Figure 8

directions along the length of the spine, from the crown of the head to the bottom of the pelvis, and across the width of the shoulders. Take three deep Alexander breaths, and release your stomach muscles. Give directions to free up the primary control (all in the manner described earlier). Now start swaying from side to side. Notice how the weight shifts from the left foot to the right foot; allow your consciousness to be fully with the sense of your body weight dropping through the soles of your feet and into the ground. Notice how the right knee bends and then the left knee bends, but in the middle both legs are straight and the weight is equally distributed. Stay with the swinging motion. Make sure that your ankles, knees and hip joints are free. Keep your *back back* and

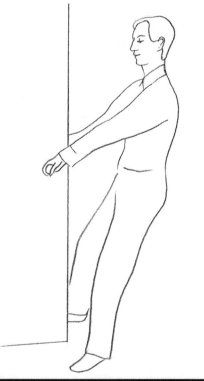

Figure 9

directions flowing along the spine. Do this for several minutes or for however long seems comfortable and enjoyable.

In this practice avoid the danger of collapsing forward from the shoulders and hollowing the chest. A slight variation of this exercise will help you to experiment with a new alignment. Look at Figure 9. The man has his feet placed fairly close to the door, wider than a shoulder's width apart, but now he holds onto a door handle and leans back until his arms are straight with no tension in the hands, arms or shoulders. Before you try out this position just make sure that you are wearing non-slip socks or bare feet and check that the door handle can safely take your weight. (If the height of the door handle is the wrong height just tie a rope around it and fix a smooth wooden handle to it a few feet away.)

Now you can try it out and feel how comfortable it is. Relax backwards and make sure that your head, neck and back are in a continuous alignment. Give directions along the length of your spine to the crown of your head, and across your shoulders, and keep your *back back*. Give directions to *allow* the primary control to be free. Keep feeling the cushion of air supporting your back from behind. Now start swinging from the left foot to the right foot and back again. It is basically the same as swinging from side to side as in Figure 8, but now you have the added advantage of being able to lean right back without fear. Continue this practice for several minutes.

When you have finished, practise walking around the room. You may well feel taller, lighter and more relaxed. You will probably also be able to stand and walk with a new postural alignment that is further back than your habitual one because the habitual compulsion has been broken by exercising in a new alignment. This is a marvellous way to start the day and I recommend all of my students to do this for several minutes first thing each morning before showering, and of course at any other time of the day when you want to realign your back.

We can now move onto the basic lunge position in Figure 10, which is a

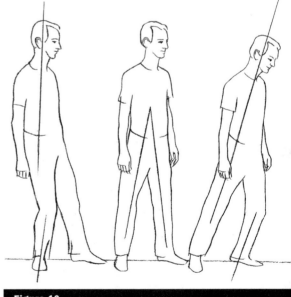

Figure 10

sequence of movements recommended by Patrick McDonald, one of Alexander's assistant teachers (who was well known for the effortless power of his directions up along the spine). The basic lunge position is shown in the middle of the sequence and it is a stronger and more stable position than having both feet parallel, where you could easily be pushed over and would have no strength to resist an attack. Here in the lunge position you widen your base by stepping forward with one foot. After that you twist the pelvis and open the front foot outwards, both about 30 degrees so that your torso is now facing in the direction of your front knee and your front foot. When you look down it now appears as if your back foot has opened out slightly by comparison. In this position you have spread your base so you can now transfer your weight from one foot to the other easily, and your centre of gravity will always be over a solid, wide base. It is now very hard to push you over with a surprise attack, and more importantly you are now in a position to release any unnecessary muscular tension at the back of your pelvis with directions and thus generate a strong flow of energy up along the spine. This is a very dynamic position because it allows for easy movement and a smooth transfer of your weight forwards or backwards, and you also have a strong back leg to twist around.

Make sure that your feet are a comfortable distance apart so that you are not hollowing your lower back, and now give directions to *allow* the widening of the lower back and a lengthening of the legs. Something like:

> "*The back of my pelvis is this wide, around the back*
> *of my pelvis to my hip joints.*
> *It is this wide and it doesn't need to be any wider*
> *or any narrower.*

I accept it just the way it is right now."

Now add directions to *allow* a lengthening of the legs:

"I am aware of the length of my legs,
from my hip joints, to my knees, to my ankles
and heels and the soles of my feet.
My legs are this long and they do not need to be
any longer or shorter,
I accept them just the way they are right now."

As you maintain these directions, say for at least 30 seconds or longer, you may suddenly become aware of a greater sense of strength and solidity in your legs as your weight releases into the ground through the soles of your feet and you experience a counter-thrust back from the ground. You may experience a sense of warmth and a sensation of the soles of your feet releasing and spreading out over the earth like the pads on an animal's feet.

The advantage of the lunge position is that it allows for this very strong sense of grounding. Now you are in a position to add directions along the length of the spine, from the crown of the head to the bottom of the pelvis, and across the width of the shoulders. Take three deep Alexander breaths, and release your stomach muscles. Give directions to free up the primary control. Keep your *back back* and keep imagining the cushion of air supporting you from behind. Now bring some movement into it: slowly transfer the weight onto the front foot as shown in Figure 10. The front knee bends but the back leg stays straight. Now shift back into the central position where both legs are straight. Shift even further back and allow the back leg to bend at the knee whilst the front leg stays straight. You will know if you have got the angle of the feet right because each time you shift your weight and bend a knee the toes should align with the movement of the knee - so that you are bending your knee directly over the line of the foot and the toes. This occurs in both the bending of your front and back leg. You should never do this exercise if the knee bending is not over the line of your foot and toes, because it will cause a twist in the knee.

Practise this exercise for several minutes just noticing how the weight shifts from one foot to another and back again. If you are practising correctly there should be a deep feeling of groundedness, and an unimpeded refreshing flow of energy from head to foot. Most importantly this exercise teaches you how to stay open with a strong flow of energy as you flow smoothly into movement. Calmly active or actively calm you can keep a feeling of inner calmness and balance at all times.

The lunge position is so basic to the Alexander Technique and so useful that we need to look at several variations of this in different applications. Firstly, it is very useful if you want a strong, solid base when you have to stand for long periods of time, eg, when talking to people at social events, when giving a speech or a presentation, or when viewing pictures at an art gallery. In all of these situations you can observe people leaning against door posts and walls, hanging onto the edge of tables and chairs or holding onto their partners as they rub their aching backs. It is not a weakness of the spine, it is simply because these people have not been taught how to stand up properly.

Now if you just review the previous lunge exercise, repeat that and then take yourself back onto the back foot and stop. Straighten the back leg and stand with about 70 per cent of your weight on that back leg. Make sure that you have first given *directions to allow the pelvis to widen across the back of the pelvis and then to allow the leg to lengthen down the length of the leg* - which is the most effective way to release the tension at the back of the pelvis.

Give directions, such as:

> *"My pelvis is this wide*
> *around the back of my pelvis to my hip joints,*
> *It is this wide and it doesn't need to be any narrower or wider.*
> *I accept it fully.*
> *It is fine the way it is right now."*

> *"My back leg is this long,*
> *from the hip joint, to the knee, to the ankle and heel,*
> *it is this long and it doesn't need to be any longer or shorter.*
> *I accept it fully the way it is right now."*

Because you do not care if that leg is lengthening or not and you fully accept yourself the way that you are right now, you relax and release, and into that release the energy of directions can now flow. The excessive muscular tension that was causing all those aches and pains in the lower back has now released and your posture is now carried by the flow of directions, which is energy. You are now standing with added strength in your legs and the pelvis feels solid and calm. The buttocks have dropped down and round. The pelvis is also completely level, because both legs are straight even though more weight is on the back leg. The spine is properly grounded in the pelvis and can now lengthen upwards where it easily supports the weight of the head. This is demonstrated in Figure 11.

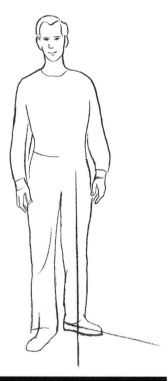

Figure 11

This is not a 'doing' - ie, trying to position the pelvis in a certain way - it is a very subtle and effortless sense of 'releasing' the excessive muscular tension through directions, which then allows the spine to lengthen and the pelvis to swing into its correct alignment relative to the balance line and the spine. If you have difficulty practising this on your own (and most people do!) then it is important to have personal Alexander Technique lessons so that your teacher can give you the hands-on experience of what it is like to release through the power of directions.

This is a very powerful position. The difference in terms of energy charge and 'presence' in the room - as compared to standing with one leg bent, the pelvis twisted and the lower back hollowed out - is like day and night. You can stand like this for a long time. You can also alternate this with the basic lunge movement that I described earlier, where you gently shift the weight onto the front foot and then onto the back foot. I remember one student of mine who came for Alexander Technique lessons. He was a biker who turned up on his Harley Davidson, a likeable young man, dressed in a leather jacket and jeans. He loved this standing position, he found it so enjoyable to stand like this at the bar with his mates, looking strong and quietly confident. Anyway, he came for a few lessons and then disappeared again, but he assured me that he had plenty of opportunity to practise this lunge standing position by standing every night in his local pub!

This is such a useful position for anyone to learn, especially an actor, public speaker or a business executive giving a presentation. As you can see in Figure 12, this position supports expressive arm movements when you need to enliven your talk or emphasise a point. More importantly you also learn how to contact yourself at a deeper level of being, in the middle of your abdomen you contact your 'centre'. The Japanese would call it 'Hara', a businessman might call it his 'gut-level response'. I would say it has a lot to do with sincerity and honesty, knowing who you

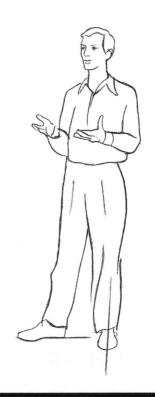

Figure 12

are and what you want and being able to communicate that honestly to the world - without holding back through fear of other people's opinions. It is a deeper level of knowing, a deeper level of being, and being honest to that and allowing it to flow out into the world through your voice, through your eyes and through your bodily gestures. There is no holding back through fear, no constricting yourself into a smaller space, no restriction of the breathing. You can expand to take up the space that is rightfully yours and give your opinion. Let your words, let your being, let your purpose flow into the world.

The most important thing about the lunge position is that the hollow in the lower back has filled out, through the use of directions,

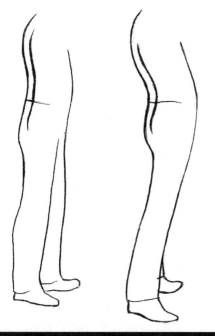

Figure 13

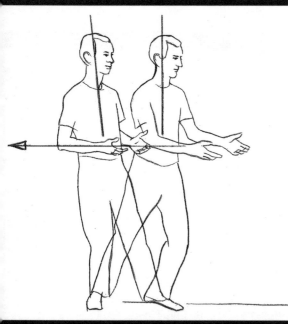

Figure 14

as demonstrated in Figure 13. The strength and stability that this gives is remarkable, but it comes from the muscular release and the inner flow of energy. To really experience the full magnitude of what this means takes many years of practice, but this process can be significantly accelerated when the direct experience can be transmitted through the hands of an experienced Alexander Technique teacher during the course of a lesson.

Now look at some more practical applications of the lunge, as in Figure 14. Here the lunge position is being used to pick up an object at waist height, eg, to pick up a book or a file from a desk. This is a whole body movement that allows the legs to do most of the work rather than just the back or arms. First pause for a moment to consider how you can get as close as possible to the desk where the book is resting. Position feet in the lunge position, with the front foot as close to the desk as possible, but allowing room for the knee to bend forwards. Now smoothly transfer the body weight onto the front foot as the body moves forwards towards the desk and hands extend to gently pick up the book from the desk top. Having grasped the book or the object, move the whole body smoothly backwards until the weight is on the back foot. There must be no jerking or snatching, just a smooth continuous movement that involves the whole of the body rather than just grabbing the object with an arm. Now you can turn to walk away carrying the object easily with your whole balance line rather than straining in an uncoordinated manner. So simple, so easy. All it takes is that little pause (inhibition) beforehand in order to organise yourself properly. This same sequence of movements can be used to open and close doors, pull and push, when vacuuming the house - the list is endless.

You might ask, "Why bother? It all seems too complicated." Well, firstly, nothing is too much bother if you are suffering from the excruciating pain of a bad back. You would do anything to try and alleviate the pain. Secondly, the advantages of the Alexander Technique are subtle and far reaching. This lunge sequence is something that involves the psycho-physical whole. Say you are opening a door using this movement pattern. You are actually integrating both your left and your right brain hemispheres in order to shift the body weight forward, grasp the door handle and then move back with it. It is a holistic movement pattern that creates new neural pathways in the brain, that links a definite cognitive purpose with a holistic awareness of your whole body movement, balance, and directions in space. It costs you a few seconds to organise yourself differently and you are moving a bit more slowly, but at the end of the procedure you are in a completely different head space, a state of 'mindfulness' as the Buddhists would say, which is a state of heightened awareness of simple everyday actions.

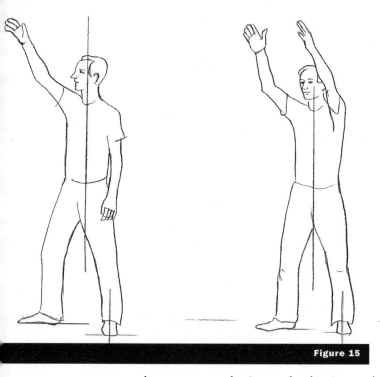

Figure 15

Let's now look at how the lunge position can support extended arm movements. Look at Figure 15 where the man could be taking an object from a high shelf or painting a room. Normally if you make a movement like that the danger is that you could raise the shoulder, stiffen the neck and hollow the back. If you are doing that all day long, or at regular intervals, that is very bad news for your shoulders. The figure in Figure 15 is actually demonstrating how to move whilst staying calm and breathing in a relaxed Alexander manner, and maintaining directions from the base of the spine up to the crown of the head, across the width of the shoulders and across the width of the pelvis. He is actually supporting his arm movements by keeping his shoulders heavy and relaxed whilst giving directions to lengthen down to the base of the spine. If you maintain these directions you can work all day without strain.

Part of the purpose of the Alexander Technique is to help you to discover new possibilities in the range of your movements. Many adults will never allow themselves to gesticulate with the full width of their arm movements. An uninhibited child will allow themselves to open their arms out wide but this is forbidden territory for most adults. So it is important to practise the bird-wing exercise in Figure 16. Standing in the lunge position for extra support from the lower back, give directions along the length of the spine, from the crown of the head to the bottom of the pelvis, and across the width of the shoulders. Allow three deep Alexander breaths, and release your stomach muscles. Give directions

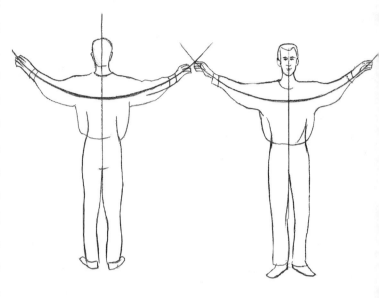

Figure 16

along the length of your neck and forward to the tip of your chin, to free up the primary control. Think that your shoulders are heavy and relaxed and allow the arms to hang loosely downwards, imagine that oil or honey is dripping down from the tips of your fingers. Now give directions to allow the arms to lengthen, such as:

> *"My arms are this long,*
> *from my shoulders, to my elbows, to my wrists,*
> *hands and the tips of my fingers.*
> *My arms are this long and I accept them completely.*
> *They are fine the way they are right now."*

Then allowing the movement to start from the tips of your fingers, lift both arms slowly to the sides (to about shoulder height) and then back down again. Keep the wrists free to allow slight movements in

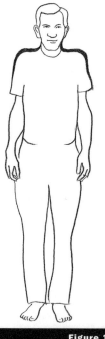

Figure 17

the hands. Feel the buoyancy in the forearms as you lift up and especially notice the pressure of the air underneath the arms and hands as you float back down again. Keep repeating this several times, making sure that you keep your shoulders heavy and relaxed. I have named this the bird-wing exercise, and it really teaches you how light and free your shoulder and arm movements can be when supported by the strength of your lower back.

The shoulders generally are one of the most problematic areas. Especially when you feel under pressure, burdened and stressed out, or if you feel insecure, fearful and under attack - up go the shoulders! Look at Figure 17 where the man is standing with hunched shoulders and a rather anxious expression on his face. Does it look familiar? It is called the 'startle response' and everyone is familiar with it. The trouble is that some people walk around like that all the time and it is generally a sign of extreme nervousness and vulnerability.

If you notice yourself doing this, the first thing to do is to physically drop the shoulders. Just tell them to relax and be heavy. The next thing to do is to stand in the lunge position for extra support from the lower back, give directions along the length of the spine, from the crown of the head to the bottom of the pelvis, and across the width of the shoulders. Allow three deep, slow Alexander breaths, and release your stomach muscles. Give directions along the length of your neck and directions along the length of the jaw bone, forwards to the tip of your chin, to free up the primary control (which is indicated by the free balance of the head on top of the spinal column). The important thing about the shoulders is to first get the vertical alignment sorted out so that there is a strong spinal column solidly grounded into a wide and spacious pelvis. Once the vertical alignment has been sorted out it should then be possible to give orders to *allow* the shoulders to widen and so to hang lightly - like a clothes hanger hooked onto a hook. This analogy is actually very accurate because the whole shoulder girdle, consisting of the two shoulder blades and the two collar bones, from which the two arms then hang at the shoulder joints, *this whole shoulder girdle literally hangs onto the rest of the skeleton at only one point.* That point is where those two funny nodules stick out at the ends of your collar bones near the bottom of your throat and fit onto your breastbone. This is the sternoclavicular joint where the collar bone (clavicle) moves on the breastbone (sternum).

Thus you can see that the shoulder girdle is literally floating in a sea of muscle, only lightly attached at one place. This means that if there is habitual over-tension of the neck and shoulder muscles the whole area can seize up like a block of concrete. Many of my students have come for precisely this problem and the only way to release this terrible pain and tension is when the shoulder girdle reconnects with the spinal column which grows out of a strong and stable pelvis. The answer to excessive shoulder tension actually lies in the pelvis! When this structure is in place the shoulder muscles are then like clothes that hang over the hanger of the shoulder girdle, loosely, lightly and easily.

The most important directions for the shoulders are to *allow* a widening across the front of the chest and across the back of the shoulders. Something like:

"I am this wide across the front of my chest,
along my collar bones and into my shoulder joints.
I am this wide across my back
from my spine across my shoulder blades and into
the shoulder joints,
to the left and to the right. I am this wide.
I don't need to be any wider or any narrower.
I accept myself totally as I am at this point in time.
I don't have to change anything because
I am perfect already."

If you don't want anything and don't expect anything this can allow some release across the width in its own time. In addition, there is the tendency for most people to also pull their arms in tightly to the body as well as hunching up the shoulders - which you can notice in Figure 17. Psychologically it is a way of appearing less threatening and less noticeable by taking up less body space. This creates a tremendous amount of unnecessary tension around the shoulder blades at the back. To counteract this tendency you will need directions to free up the shoulder blades, such as:

"I am aware of a line from the bottom tip of my
shoulder blade down to my pelvic girdle.
There is this much distance between my shoulder
blade and my pelvis.
It doesn't need to be more or less.
I accept this space exactly as it is right now."

With unlimited time and without any expectations of anything this will release into a slight natural forward curve and a widening of the shoulder blades. There can also be a sense of the space between the shoulder blades and the pelvis coming alive so that the shoulders feel supported by the ribcage and the pelvis below them. To maintain this release it is now necessary to give directions from the shoulders down to the elbows, with a slight outward direction at the elbows so that you keep some air space between the inside of your arms and the ribcage. Something like:

"I am aware of the distance between
my shoulder joint and my elbow.
It doesn't need to be any longer or shorter.
I accept it just the way it is right now."

"I am aware that my elbows are pointing
out slightly to either side.
I am aware of the air space between
the inside of my arms and my ribcage.
I accept it just the way it is right now."

As you can see from Figure 18, the position of the arms and shoulders has significantly changed as a result of giving directions, and as a psycho-physical being this new posture will also be reflected in a more open and self-confident mental and emotional state. However, the illustration can only give a very superficial impression of the change and cannot at all describe the complex series of directions that led to this transformation.

When lifting and carrying any object it is important to work with the basic Alexander principles as illustrated in Figure 19.

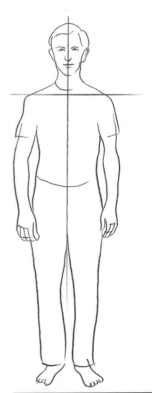

Figure 18

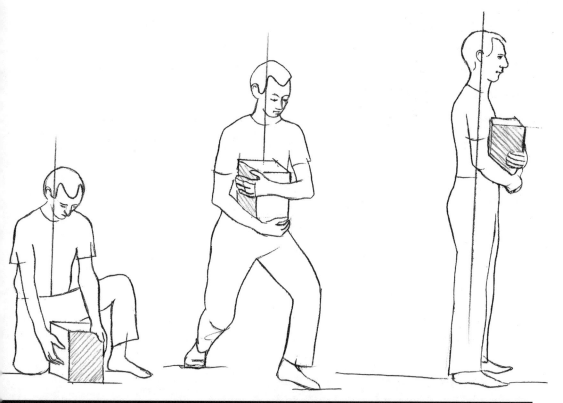

Figure 19

These basic principles are:

(1)   Carry the weight as close as possible to your centre
of gravity.

(2)   When lifting, work using the knees and hips,
allowing your legs to do the work without straining
your back or shoulders.

(3)   Keep an awareness of your balance and give directions
from the crown of your head down to your ankles,
heels and the soles of your feet to *allow* a lengthening
to take place.

As you can see in Figure 19 the man is about to lift a heavy object up from the ground. The first thing to do is to *pause* and consider how to position yourself as close as possible to the object so as not to make a sudden, jerky lifting movement that could strain the back. Go down on one knee if possible. (If your knees hurt use a modified lunge position where your back heel is slightly off the ground, as demonstrated by the position of the feet in the middle of the sequence in figure 19.) The important thing is that you are as close to the object as possible so that you can get your hands underneath it, keeping the arms straight and the back aligned. Lift the box onto one thigh, then holding it close to your chest straighten your legs, so that you are lifting the object using your powerful leg muscles rather than straining your back. Stand comfortably in your balance line, continuing to give directions, and then walk away.

Practising standing and sitting using the Alexander Technique is something that you will find yourself doing a lot of during the course of your Alexander lessons. This is not because standing and sitting is terribly important in itself, it is more a convenient opportunity for your teacher to help you to spot where you are stiffening and holding at certain critical points of the sequence, and to help you to correct these bad habits through the use of directions. The whole point is to stay perfectly balanced over your heels at all stages of this smooth-flowing sequence - so that if someone were to suddenly take away the chair you would not fall over! It is also surprising how little effort is needed in order to stand up or sit down when your directions are flowing - it is as if the movement does itself.

Look at Figure 20. Starting from a standing position with the feet parallel and about a shoulder's width apart, and remaining completely unconcerned about the end goal of getting your bottom

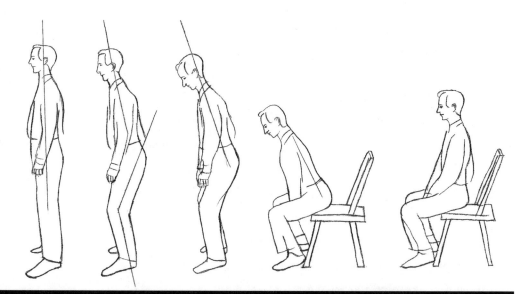

Figure 20

onto a chair, start to give directions. Give directions along the length of the spine, from the crown of the head to the soles of the feet (making sure that you have slightly more weight on your heels than on the balls of your feet), and across the width of the shoulders. *Allow* three deep Alexander breaths to flow in and out, and release your stomach muscles. Give directions along the length of your neck and along the jaw bone to the tip of your chin, to free up the primary control. Think that your shoulders are heavy and relaxed and allow the arms to hang loosely downwards.

Start by bending the knees and the hips, keeping your body weight balanced over your heels. About halfway down check to see if you have stiffened your neck and pulled your head back and down in an effort to maintain eye contact whilst talking to other people in the room. If you have made this classic mistake *pause for a bit* and *very slightly tuck your chin in* as you can see the man doing in the third picture of the sequence. This helps you to keep the muscles along the nape of the neck lengthened. The eyes are now looking slightly downwards to the floor rather than straight ahead into the room. This is only done as a preventative measure to stop you pulling your head back and down and shortening your neck muscles unnecessarily. Then continue to parachute down slowly until you land lightly on the edge of the chair. Now swing the torso back from the hip joints until you end up in an upright, balanced sitting posture with the eyes looking forwards. Notice how during this whole sequence the head/neck/back relationship has functioned as one living unit, rather than being broken at some point through a collapse and a rounding of the back, which would cut off the flow of energy.

Whilst in the balanced sitting position continue to give directions to *allow the neck to be free, to let the head go forward and up, to let the back lengthen and widen. Continue to give directions from the crown of the head right down to the base of the spine as you sit balanced on your sitting bones (at the bottom of your pelvis).*

Standing up is almost exactly the reverse sequence of sitting down *except that you can start by just slightly dropping your chin.* Once again, this is only a preventative measure to stop the classic mistake of tightening your neck muscles and pulling your head back and down as a sort of muscular bracing preparatory to standing up. Now swivel forwards from the hips until your centre of gravity is over your heels and push downwards with your heels into the ground in order to stand up. Keep your *'back back'*, by sensing a cushion of air behind your back at all times. Make sure that your eyes continue to look towards the floor at a downwards angle until your knees have straightened and you are standing up straight. The main point of this exercise is to avoid the tendency to tighten muscles unnecessarily at several critical stages of this sequence. It is surprising how little muscular effort is needed when you are working with the primary control and getting the upthrust from the ground through your heels at all times. The body seems to float up and parachute down rather than be forced by will-power and muscular effort. Once again you are going with the flow rather than using excessive (and habitual!) muscular tension.

Walking is something that we all do everyday and, regardless of whether it is performed as a form of pleasant outdoor exercise, or simply to get from A to B, walking should be done with a balanced, upright posture. You can have a feeling of gliding through space calmly aware of the beauty of the moment and the scenery around you rather than rushing ahead of yourself, both mentally and physically, so as to arrive at your destination more quickly.

The first prerequisite is to consciously discover your balance line, so repeat the balance exercise swaying backwards and forwards from

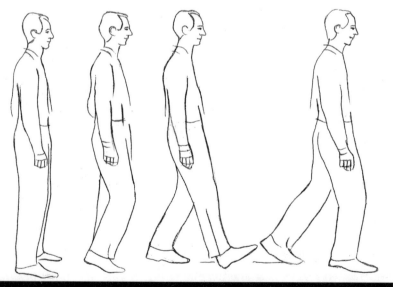

Figure 21

your heels until you finally come to rest in a position of perfect equilibrium. Give directions from the crown of your head down to your ankles and heels to *allow* your back to lengthen, and across the width of your shoulders. Give directions along the length of your neck to *allow* the neck to be free, and also forward to the tip of your chin. Give directions to *allow* the back of your pelvis to widen, and then along the length of your legs down to the ankles and heels to *allow* your legs to lengthen.

Now start walking in a perfectly natural manner as shown in Figure 21, but pay attention to three things. Firstly, keep your *back back* in this new alignment by visualising a cushion of air behind you. If you find yourself reverting back to your old habitual style of walking (perhaps by leaning forwards too much with rounded shoulders) just say, "No" and stop everything for a moment. Come back to your balance line with the swaying exercise and then start walking again. If you have ever been to India and seen those beautiful peasant woman walking back from the well with a heavy pot of water balanced on their heads you will know what I mean. They just seem to glide forward through space so effortlessly and elegantly. The heavy weight of the water is exactly aligned with their centre of gravity and their balance line as they walk. As you can see in the second figure along, the man bends his knee to lift his leg but his back stays back in the optimal alignment.

Secondly, as you put your front foot forward make sure that you contact the ground very definitely with your heel first. Notice how the third man along is putting his front foot down with the heel first. At the same time his back heel is just beginning to peel off the ground. As he continues with his forward momentum in the fourth figure almost all of his weight has been transferred to his front foot (which is now fully on the ground) whilst only the toes of his back foot remain in contact with the ground. So the back of your heel should contact the ground first and you then roll onto the ball of your foot and toes. It is heel-toe, heel-toe the whole time as you are walking.

Thirdly, keep your stomach soft and relaxed and your breathing deep and calm. Try to keep your attention on being in the moment, rather than on your memories of the past or hopes and fears for the future. Paying attention to the rhythm of your breath will bring you into the present moment. Enjoy the scenery around you, enjoy the feeling of being alive and outdoors, breathing fresh air and getting fresh oxygen and life energy into your system.

You should walk until the mind feels calm and serene and you can feel yourself settling into an easy, natural rhythm of movement - which generally takes about 20-30 minutes. Experiment with different speeds and aim to practise every day. Walking is one of the best forms of exercise but to get the most benefit from it you should also be using the Alexander Technique at the same time. It is also very clever to have a specific everyday activity - like walking - when you deliberately practise the Alexander Technique at the same time.

Of the greatest help in the release of over-tensed muscles and the realignment of the spine is the regular practice of lying down flat on your back in the semi-supine position. This should be done after lunch for 10-15 minutes and again in the early evening or before going to bed. When lying in the semi-supine position you can relax your muscles completely because gravity is no longer a problem, and you can also relax your mind by paying attention to your breathing pattern. The great advantage of the semi-supine is that it takes the weight-bearing pressure off your spine and allows the intervertebral discs to reabsorb fluid and thus regain their size and shape.

It releases aches and pains and you can regenerate your energy and mental focus in a very short space of time.

In Figure 22 you can see the semi-supine position demonstrated. Notice that the knees are up, the hands are resting on top of the pelvis, palms down, and the head is resting

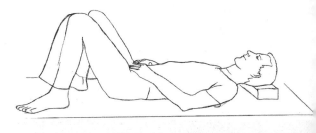

Figure 22

on top of a book. The height of the book is very important because it supports the head so that the neck vertebrae lie parallel to the ground and are not under any strain. You can lie on the carpet on the floor, or on a table covered with a blanket, but only lie on a bed if it has a very firm orthopaedic mattress. The advantages of the semi-supine are obvious: it is as if you are lying on a large ironing board and gravity is straightening out your spinal vertebrae. But first it is necessary to make two small adjustments to completely flatten out the spine.

The first adjustment is demonstrated in Figures 23-26. This shows you how to flatten out your lower back on your own. First press your feet down and lift your pelvis off the ground as in Figure 23. Next place your hands, palms up, near the top of your pelvis and *slowly* start to run your hands down over your buttocks, as in Figure 24 to slightly alter the tilt of your pelvis. As the palms of your hands continue to *slowly* rub down over your buttocks start to allow the lower spinal vertebrae to drop back gently onto the ground, one by one, like the pearls of a necklace dropping into place: click, click, click. You can see in Figure 25 that the top lumbar vertebrae are already down. Finally, it is only the coccyx that needs to be tilted round slightly and then dropped back down, as in Figure 26. There

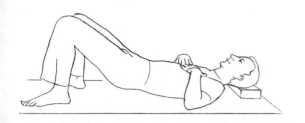

Figure 23

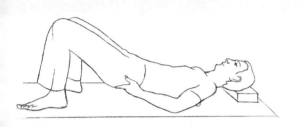

Figure 24

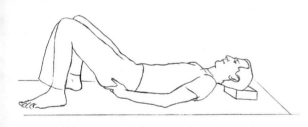

Figure 25

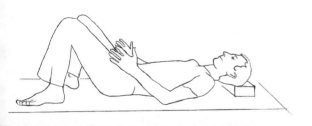

Figure 26

is a definite progression to this sequence and it needs to be done slowly and deliberately. There is no point in rushing it. Your lower back should now be completely flat against the ground with no hollow at all. There is often an immediate feeling of release and relaxation.

The second adjustment involves straightening out the neck. Place your hands as in Figure 27 so that you can hold the weight of your head and just gently tilt it forwards and pull it outwards very slightly at the same time to straighten the neck vertebrae and release the neck muscles. Place your head back on the book again in this new position. Close your eyes and relax, as in Figure 28. Notice the difference. Through these two subtle adjustments you now have a gentle stretch working throughout the whole length of your spine. Even if you do nothing else except lie there and have a short catnap for 10 minutes, your back will be relaxing and realigning itself through the power of that stretch.

Of course I would prefer it if you don't go to sleep because you will get far more benefit from these 10-15 minutes if you lie there and watch your breath and give directions. Now you are ready to begin. First switch off your mind from all worries and distractions. This time is for you to utilise for positive regeneration. Get into a pattern of deep, calm Alexander breathing, as described in the section on breathing (p. 52). Each time you breathe out allow your body to release downwards onto the ground, allow a little bit of tension to just flow into the ground and

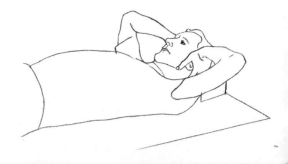

Figure 27

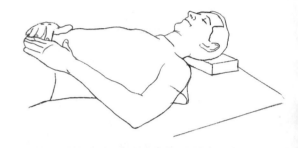

Figure 28

disappear. *Allow* the inhalation to flow in by itself without any effort on your part. Any effort used should only be to make sure that all the air is expelled from your lungs. After a time do nothing at all, just keep watching the ebb and flow of your breath in a very detached manner, without trying to control it. Just be aware of it and every time you breathe out just relax your back, back down onto the table.

Start to give directions along the length of your spine from the crown of your head down to the base of your spine. Give directions across the width of your shoulders. Give directions to *allow* your neck to be free.

A good way of releasing the neck is to visualise that the back of the neck is supported by soft, warm sand, or a hot-water bottle, or feathers, or cotton wool, or a cushion of air, or whatever works for you. This is often best done when lying down on your back where you can talk to your neck muscles and say:

"Look, you are on holiday now, there is no work for you to do so you can relax and take it easy. The soft sand along the nape of my neck and at the back of my head is supporting all the weight of my head and neck. I feel supported, I feel safe, my neck muscles can relax and do less and less."

Use whatever visualisation works for you and talk to your neck muscles in this way. After you get up into a vertical position imagine there is a cushion of air behind your neck, supporting and releasing your neck muscles. It works, because the mind can convince the body of the reality of any idea.

At the same time you have to be giving directions to release the jaw muscles. These are some of the most powerful muscles in the body and if you try deliberately tensing your jaw muscles now you will see how that automatically tenses the back of your neck. As you release, the neck releases. So to release further you need to think a line along the jaw to the tip of the chin, and say to yourself:

"My jaw is this far forwards,
it doesn't need to be further forwards
or further retracted.
I accept it,
it is fine the way it is right now."

Repeat this direction and hold the thought for at least 30 seconds, whilst you keep thinking directions to free the neck at the same time. Because the neck is releasing backwards whilst the jaw is releasing forwards you may have created a tiny gap in the middle, a bit more space, a sense of balanced release at the atlanto-occipital joint where the head balances on top of the spinal column. This is a very precise point and a subtle opening takes place here. Even if you do not have this sense of an opening at the beginning, you can still think a direction from the crown of the head down to the base of the spine, and the direction will flow because it isn't blocked at the top joint. So you can *'let the back lengthen and widen'* by thinking directions along the length, until the spine feels firmly grounded in the pelvis, and across the width to *'allow'* the shoulders and pelvis to widen.

Continue to lie on the table or the ground for a full 10-15 minutes feeling your back releasing backwards into the ground, *allowing* it to lengthen and widen so that it is getting flatter and spreading out like a pancake. Think directions to:

> *"allow the arms to lengthen*
> *from the shoulder joints to the tips of the fingers,"*

and

> *"allow the legs to lengthen*
> *from the hip joints down to the ankles and heels,*
> *the soles of the feet and the tips of the toes."*

After you have relaxed the body and calmed the mind it is time to think about how to get up correctly. You should certainly not jerk the body up into a sitting position and tense the neck muscles all over again as that ruins everything! The correct sequence is shown in Figures 29-31. You start by rolling over onto your side as in Figure 29. Make sure that you lie fully on the down shoulder with

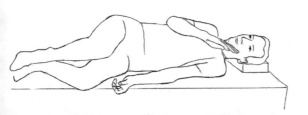

Figure 29

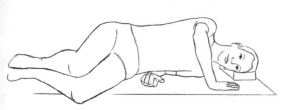

Figure 30

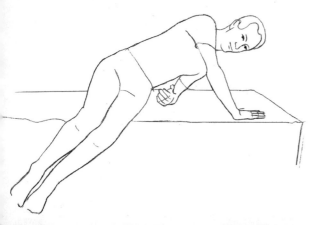

Figure 31

the elbow of your lower arm tucked under your body, as shown in Figure 30. Then push yourself up into a sitting position using your top arm and the elbow of your lower arm for support, keeping the spine straight, as demonstrated in Figure 31. (This smooth, easy sequence is also the way you should get up out of bed, especially if you have back problems.) Once you get up from the semi-supine notice how you feel more relaxed and how your alignment has improved.

Chapter 7

THE PSYCHOLOGICAL SIGNIFICANCE OF POSTURE

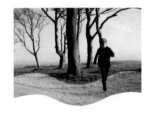

WHO AM I?

I f you are a careful observer of people around you, on the tube, in supermarkets, on the street, in the theatre, at parties, or wherever, you will be amazed at the sheer diversity of human movement and posture. If you then pause for a while and actually try to imitate and feel what it is like to be inside that other person, you will be surprised at the insights you can gain and you will probably end up feeling very happy to be you rather than them. This can be a useful exercise, so long as we don't get stuck in judgements of others whilst remaining blind to our own faults.

Body language is something many of us have become familiar with recently, especially since certain sections of the tabloid press have arranged for psychologists to analyse the postures of certain renowned personalities. Sadly, however, the purpose of this analysis is commercial and destructive rather than being in any way therapeutic and transformative. What, however, are the most obvious variations in posture that we can notice? Firstly, the carriage of the head and the way the eyes and the line of the jaw go out to meet the world. If there is an alertness, a freshness and buoyancy (which we in the Alexander world would describe as the 'forward and up') to the face and head then this projects a most refreshing and enlivening influence onto the immediate environment. Conversely, someone who hangs their head low refusing to meet your gaze and seems to be sunk into themselves, creates an impression of dejection, depression and defeat. Are you one of life's losers or one of life's conquerors? Your posture reveals all! We can all contact that spirit deep within which transcends any possibility of defeat despite the most appalling outer difficulties confronting us. Connected with this, the precondition for the head being light and Up is the release of the throat and neck muscles. This is something that isn't particularly noticeable to the casual observer but is immediately perceptible to anyone with experience of the Alexander Technique. A stiff neck denotes dogmatism, fixation and inflexibility of the type associated with the phrase 'keep a stiff upper lip' or a 'redneck'. Such a neck, like a brittle tree on a mountainside, will break if exposed to a wind of any strength. A free and flexible neck on the other hand is a sign of openness, an ability to react spontaneously in response to the situation as it is. There is a wonderful calmness and tolerance in a free neck which, like the stem of a supple tree on a mountainside, can bend with even the most powerful wind, and cannot be broken.

The Significance of Posture

The **back of the neck** is part of the bridge that connects the abstract, mental head with the physical reality of our bodies and emotional reactions. There is a tremendous sensitivity here as this part of the body has one of the highest concentrations of sensory nerve endings. And yet due to habitual patterns of tension many people are not even aware that they have a stiff neck, and are blocking off all the information about their shoulders, back and pelvis - information that a free neck would naturally be giving them. In a sense the back of the neck relates to the past, and a confidence and stability based on past achievements and experiences. We have something behind us that enables us to maintain our position in relation to other people and the world in general through a strong, erect spine, but it is a quiet strength based on inner self-confidence and independence. There is balance. If we can feel a quality of strength behind us, why do we need to come forward to demand or beg from others, and to suffer possible disappointments and frustrations? An individual who is balanced between the forward and back will not have to beg from a position of neediness, but can ask from a position of strength.

The **throat,** like the neck, is part of the narrow bridge connecting the head with the rest of the body, and due to its tightness this gorge can easily get blocked with the debris of past experiences. Through the mouth and throat we have to take in food, liquids and air, so it is one of the main areas of intake for the body and a blockage there can indicate a refusal to 'swallow' the symbolic food of other people's ideas or views about reality. At some deep level we are aware when we are being fed rubbish and yet we may not have the courage or insight to express and maintain our alternative point of view. How many times as children have we been forced to 'eat our words' and retract a statement that the adult world found unacceptable? Obviously the throat is our organ of speech, the means by which we express our thoughts and emotions, so our inhibitions and judgements about what is or isn't appropriate to express can set up powerful conflicts and tensions that naturally will be manifested in the throat itself.

The **front part of the throat** in a sense relates to our ability to release our creative word into the world. It is perhaps the most innovative part of the human body in that thoughts, feelings and aspirations issuing from our innermost core are released here into the flow of the space-time continuum, to germinate, grow and have an effect upon our world. Now, if we are not really sure who we are or what our real role in life is, or if we have doubts and fears about how our words will be received, then there will be a feeling of tightness in the throat, the larynx will be depressed and the jaw pulled back into the throat. The words may never actually get spoken, or if they are they will come out half-heartedly or aggressively to cover up our inner doubt and confusion. When the front part of the throat begins to release, to soften and lengthen, we begin to reconnect with information coming to us from the front part of the chest, solar plexus, stomach and pelvic areas. We become free to speak our truth and to allow those words to work in the world, not because we necessarily expect others to agree with us and do it our way, but because we need to express ourselves. Truth and sincerity are powers in themselves that will work in the world irrespective of whether others wish to listen or not at this point in time.

The **spine** is quite literally the backbone of our being. It represents the column of the skeletal system upon which everything else hangs. It can appear to be weak and disjointed, giving the impression of 'spinelessness'; nonetheless its importance cannot be overemphasised. The Alexander Technique stresses the necessity of being able to rely on the central alignment of the spine, and the feeling of the head balancing freely on top of the spinal column at the atlanto-occipital joint. The entire emphasis of the Technique has always been: go back to basics; get aligned, feel the whole length of the spine and allow all muscles (in particular those in the throat and neck regions) to relax and melt downwards with the force of gravity, hanging over the framework of the skeleton. This creates a wonderful sense of balance and calmness in the body. And because the spine houses the centres of higher spiritual perception, by linking up in this way we are also opening ourselves up to spiritual help, guidance and protection.

In the central hollow part of the spine we are connected to all aspects of our being through the sensory and motor neurons of the central nervous system, and also to the central blood supply which runs from the brain to the rest of the body. In this way every thought, feeling, event and response is impregnated in the spine as well as the relevant parts of the body. By working on the spine itself it is possible to change deeply ingrained habit patterns. And by recalling that sense of freedom under stressful conditions it is possible to maintain our ability to make conscious decisions rather than be the victims of habit or circumstance.

During the course of an Alexander lesson the student becomes aware of the flow of energy through the spine, which is actually a two-way flow from the medulla oblongata down to the coccyx region where it reverses and rises up again, realigning the stability and strength of the lower back/pelvis region with the grace and flexibility of the upper body, allowing the head to 'float' freely at the top atlanto-occipital joint.

The next thing to notice is the carriage of the **shoulders**. Many people walk around with the shoulders hunched and rounded as if they were overwhelmed by problems, as if the burden of life is too great and overwhelming. Or it can be a reaction of fright, as if living in a permanent state of shock or fear. They are giving off a very clear message which says, "Please don't come near me. I'm frightened and I don't want to talk to you." Whereas someone who allows their shoulders to widen and slot down with the natural force of gravity, stands open and relaxed and is not afraid to let the world in and communicate spontaneously with others. Hunched shoulders are a sign that you expect to be beaten, possibly from behind and unexpectedly - an expectation that may well be fulfilled if it is strongly established. There are some people who try to overcompensate for this by adopting a macho, broad-chested swagger. Body builders often do this and, whilst it may have certain advantages, it is not a balanced position, as the pinching of the vertebrae between the shoulder blades and the increased tightness of the lower back reveals. So what we are really looking for is a natural balanced openness in the shoulders - a surprisingly rare discovery.

The shoulders also represent the innermost aspect of our doing energy: are we doing what we really want to be doing in life? Are we putting our ideas into action through our shoulders, arms and hands? Are we expressing our feelings of love and caring from the heart which would like to find expression in hugging or being close to someone we love? If the answer to any of these is no, then the shoulders will tend to be stiff and tight, hollowing out the front of the chest as we close in on ourselves. The closer we keep these feelings and conflicts to ourselves, the more tense and rigid our shoulders will be. It is only as we learn how to participate more fully in life and express who we really are without fear, that the shoulders will begin to unlock and our creative impulses will flow through into our arms and hands.

Pain or tension in the upper part of the back and shoulders is likewise connected with rage and frustration at not doing what we really want to be doing, in not achieving what we really want to achieve. It is only as we begin to acknowledge what these hidden ambitions and aspirations are and to express these either in terms of our career, relationships, or spiritual yearnings, that these tension patterns will begin to dissolve.

The **arms and hands** show how we reach out to express ourselves in the world and accomplish our tasks. The classic defensive position with the arms folded on the chest indicates a closed attitude and solves the problem of what to do with your arms; whereas someone who is very expressive and enthusiastic will make large, powerful open gestures with their arms. It is very interesting to see a speeded-up film of the way children and adults move and gesticulate, for it soon becomes apparent that both groups are making basically the same gestures, but the adults generally cut themselves off short, whereas the children allow themselves the full, uninhibited expression of that gesture. On average, adults only allow themselves to go five per cent of the distance that children go, so just imagine how much potential emotion and enthusiasm is being held back! The full width of the human body, the sense of broadness and rounded space, is rarely experienced. All too often you see people going into a tall tightness, and it is so relaxing to see a nice, wide, happy, open body, that gives full expression to its width.

The hands show our ability to work, to reach out to the world and accomplish something, and we would be virtually powerless if we could not express ourselves through these tools. The quality of a person's handshake, the temperature and texture of their hand, will tell you a lot about them. Cold hands are a sign of pulling the emotional energy back into the body, and an unwillingness to come into contact with the world, to feel, to work and shape it according to our design. It can also mean a reluctance or fear to reach out in an expression of love and caring. Sweaty hands are generally a sign of nervousness and lack of self-confidence, whereas dry, warm hands are an indication of a capable person who can get a grip on things and handle their job or life's challenges in a reasonably confident and efficient manner. Allowing our fingers to be warm and alive and the entire hands to fill up with energy is one way of changing the quality of our hands. But above all we have to be capable of touching and being touched, of exposing our vulnerabilities and expressing and receiving love and tenderness.

Breathing, posture and the emotions are all inextricably linked and careful observation of the movements of the **ribcage, diaphragm and stomach muscles** tells us a great deal about a person's emotional state and the rhythmic quality of their breathing. Someone who breathes shallowly from the top of the chest is quite passive, stressful and afraid. They cannot give themselves room to express their full potential because they are imprisoned within their own, or other people's, limited expectations and judgements of them. Very often the tone of voice will sound pinched and squeezed. On the other hand, people who breathe and talk from deep down, connected to a relaxed stomach and allowing the ribcage to expand easily (because they are not trying to control the breath), are giving themselves more space and enabling themselves to contact their inner potential and influence the world from their centre - a place of quiet power and conviction. In talking or singing the voice has much more resonance and depth to it, and becomes both very personal and universal at the same time.

The **middle back,** or the area behind the solar plexus, is often an area that can get out of balance due to tightness, which can lead to the vertebrae being pulled out of alignment. This is because we are receiving so many messages from others (on an unspoken energetic level) through the solar plexus, that we frequently allow ourselves to be pulled into power struggles as we try to discover ourselves and maintain our position in the world. When confronted with hostility, people will often say, "It feels as though I've been kicked in the stomach." Or alternatively when feeling particularly focused and clear you can experience a radiation of powerful energy coming out of the solar plexus. The ideal is obviously to be so in balance that there are no hidden desires or expectations that can be manipulated by another person, and no desires of our own to have power over or to manipulate others.

The most central area of the body is the **pelvis**, where the bowels and the reproductive organs are housed. The tension patterns and tilt of the pelvis can tell us a lot about a person's attitude towards their deeper instinctual nature, and the degree to which they are in touch with their inner power. You can often see people walking around in a sort of slouch with rounded shoulders, the head and neck sunk forward, whilst there is also an exaggerated hollow in the lower back because the tail end of the pelvis is tipped up, whilst the frontal genital area points down and away to the degree that it becomes distant and disconnected from the rest of the body. The back is effectively broken in two places, and what many such people don't realise is just how disconnected and powerless they appear as they float around in a kind of 'limbo'. It is the typical slouch of the teenage rebel, the drop-out, yet sometimes it continues way beyond that time indicating a person who has grave difficulties in adjusting to the demands of life and new responsibilities. The posture has to be corrected at two places simultaneously, and the priority is actually on correcting the tilt of the pelvis, so as to ground the person, bringing them back into contact with the earth and giving them more stamina and endurance. Someone who is grounded firmly in their pelvis - with the hollow in the lower back nearly filled out, hips nice and wide, the back of the pelvis rounded with the tail tucked under, stomach muscles relaxed so that the front of the pelvis is soft and rounded down to the genitals - gives off an impression of vitality, calmness and centredness that cannot be denied.

The **lower back**, which runs down behind the solar plexus region to the coccyx, is an area representing our relationships. Fears and conflicts in personal, family and social relationships, based generally on a lack of inner security or sense of self-worth, will manifest here in tension and tightness. The base of the pelvis and the feet are areas of grounding, so that, paradoxically, fears about our ability to survive and maintain our position in the world will actually cause us to tighten the muscles at the back of the pelvis and pull up and away from the very ground we stand on, thus causing us to have even less sense of security. Conflicts with our sexual energy and the way we express, suppress, or transform that energy will also be mirrored in tension patterns in the pelvis.

The **legs** - our physical contact with the earth - give us the physical strength and vitality to move against the force of gravity. Continual crossing of the legs is quite a bad habit because it tilts the pelvis up on one side and tends to constrict the muscles around the hip joint on the same side. It is much more stable and reassuring to sit with both feet on the ground, with the body weight equally distributed through the sitting bones on each side of the pelvis and through the feet. When some people are standing you can often see that they are tensing the muscles connecting the buttocks and lower back with the thighs, and this pattern of tension actually continues all the way down behind the knees, calf muscles and ankles. If we wish to be truly grounded, it is precisely these muscles which need to be lengthening and softening so as to allow the hip joint, knees and ankles to release, thereby enabling the soles of the feet and especially the heels to ground themselves into the earth. Only then do we experience the counter-thrust of the anti-gravitational reflexes (or earth energy streams), which give the legs a feeling of lightness, strength and flexibility. We need to get rid of fear and the subconscious idea that we must tense in order to maintain our position in the world. If we go with the flow we can experience real lightness, ease, and the ability to regenerate ourselves in trying situations. Humility brings us closer to the ground, but it is also an attitude of mind that realises, "I can of myself do nothing. There is a certain openness that is my responsibility, yes, an openness to the flow which alone brings balance and ease to my life."

The **feet**, and in particular the soles of the feet, are a very special part of the body. It is important to get the feeling of the whole of the foot coming into contact with the ground. Curling up the toes and pulling them into the foot is quite common and is part of the fear reflex, a preparation for fight or flight. We need to be able to release and separate the toes from the front of the foot so there is a true lengthening and coming into contact with the ground, so we can feel sure of our way forward. Close observation will also reveal either a tendency to put too much weight on the outside edges of the feet, thus exaggerating the inner arch of the foot and leading to a very clearly defined sense of separation of self from the not-self; or else flat-footedness which is indicative of everything merging together, self and not-self, work and leisure, what I need to get done as opposed to demands on my time, etc. There are also those people who walk too far forward on the balls of the feet and toes, hardly putting any weight onto their heels at all. This prevents them from effectively grounding themselves and coming fully into contact with the ground: the reality of their situation. A natural and balanced distribution of weight on the sole of the foot takes place when the body weight passes down through the centre of gravity and into the ground, which is much further back towards the heel than we normally assume, and certainly not the middle of the foot.

General Affirmations For Releasing Tension In Different Parts of the Body

These are just some of the affirmations for different body parts that I have noted down after working with clients in my practice over many years. The list is potentially endless. Because each person is unique it is obviously better to work with an Alexander teacher experienced in psycho-physical therapy and your unique tailor-made affirmation will emerge from your Body Wisdom during the course of a session. If you cannot make the time for a personal session then the next best thing is to read through the list and choose the affirmations that particularly resonate with you. Remember the basic principle of the Alexander Technique which says that 'Primary Control' (or a sense of release throughout the whole body) can only occur when we:

> "*allow the neck to be free,*
> *allow the head to be lightly balanced on top of the*
> *spinal column,*
> *allow the back to lengthen,*
> *allow the shoulders to widen,*
> *allow the pelvis to be solidly grounded and widened.*"

That is to say, you cannot release an individual part without connecting to a total pattern of release throughout the whole body. So choose the affirmations from the list that resonate for you, choosing *at least one* from the section for the neck, the head, the back, the shoulders and the pelvis and any others that are important for you. String them all together and memorise them so that you can mentally repeat them to yourself. After each repetition pause for a few seconds to allow the affirmation to sink down from your head into your body and to impregnate your subconscious mind. Then repeat again. Repeat your affirmation at any quiet opportunity, preferably for several minutes at a time. Never try to force a result because it will just lead to further tension. *Allow releases to occur in their own time* and let the mental affirmation do the work - not the muscles!

In the head:

My head is light and clear

My head is mobile

My mind is clear and focused

My head is bright

My head feels light and balanced

In the jaw:

My jaw is soft and smooth

My jaw is released

I feel free to express myself

In the neck:

My neck is free

My neck is released

My neck is open

My neck is fat and chunky

My neck is relaxed

In the shoulders:

My shoulders feel soft and relaxed

My shoulders feel wide and strong

The top of my chest feels flat and wide

My shoulders feel open

My shoulders feel heavy and released

My shoulders feel relaxed

My shoulders are wide and have dropped back

I'm free

I'm happy

I am saying "YES" to life

I am quietly confident

I am open to the world

I feel full and rounded

In the back:

My back feels lengthened

My back feels flatter

My back feels released

My back feels stronger

In the arms and hands:

I feel energy tingling in my shoulders, arms and hands

I'm ready to get on with things

My hands feel like playing

In the heart:

My heart is open

My heart feels joyous

In the stomach:

My stomach is smooth and flowing

My stomach is settled

My stomach is relaxed

In the pelvis:

> *My pelvis feels strong and stable*
>
> *I am solid, I am stable*
>
> *I feel deeply grounded within my pelvis*
>
> *My pelvis feels warm*
>
> *I have energy in my pelvis*
>
> *My pelvis feels wide and stable*
>
> *My pelvis feels relaxed*
>
> *I have a right to exist*

In the legs and feet:

> *I feel connected to my legs and feet*
>
> *My heels are drilling down through the floor*
>
> *I can stand up for myself*

Breathing:

> *My breathing is deep and relaxed*
>
> *My breathing is even*
>
> *My breath is soft and flowing*
>
> *My breathing is calm and relaxed*

Wholeness and integration:

> *I am melting into freedom*
>
> *I feel connected to all of myself*
>
> *I have a sense of being rather than doing*
>
> *I have an intangible sense of faith and trust in life*
>
> *All the pieces of the jigsaw puzzle are clicking into place*
>
> *I feel calm and relaxed*
>
> *Energy is flowing through my entire body*
>
> *Everything is flowing*

I'm living in the moment
I'm spacious, I'm light, I'm hopeful
I feel connected to myself
I feel at ease with myself
I feel joyous
I'm a whole person
I'm liberated
I'm confident
I can handle it
I'm optimistic
I am a child of the Universe.
All good can come to me.
Everything will be all right
I feel safe and worthy and protected

RESISTANCE TO POSTURAL CHANGE

After a few lessons in the Alexander Technique the student may begin to get tantalising glimpses of the possibilities of transformation, of what it is like to be free and open with the head balanced on top of the spinal column and the back lengthening and widening. Most importantly they should have been shown what their own particular pattern of tension is and what the specific direction of release is, so that the blockage can melt and re-establish contact with other body parts, thus allowing a free flow of energy and a greater sense of cooperation and integration.

Now very often it is precisely this sense of freedom and openness that can appear intimidating to the student. The question suddenly arises: Well, if I'm not my mannerisms, if I'm not my past conditioning, if I'm not a particular way of thinking or reacting, then who on earth am I? This is a very important question. Regardless of whether it has been posed consciously or unconsciously the immediate reaction is often fear, which causes us to pull back into the old and familiar style of being. This is what I'm like, this is the way my friends and partner have always known me, and this is the way I'll stay. It would be very unsettling for everybody if I were suddenly to become something different, wouldn't it? This fear of change can present quite a formidable barrier between the tried and tested, the familiar, and the new that is striving to come into being and to release the hero/ine within us, nearing the ultimate integration and fulfilment of knowing what role we should be playing on the stage of existence, and playing it perfectly and effortlessly (because we are detached from identification with the dualities of success or failure). Yet if we think about it, since life is essentially a river of change, a continuous process of becoming, we would do well to become aware of the patterns of our thought and emotional reactions, so that we can change them and attune ourselves with Life's Flow, its ongoing process of inner and outer transformation, rather than resisting it and getting stuck in our frustration and discontent.

During the course of an Alexander Technique lesson we are constantly endeavouring to do less and less, and to let go of more and more. It is like peeling off the layers of an onion: Well, I'm not this tension pattern, so melt it away; I'm not this stiff posture, so drop it; I'm not this particular habit of reaction, so forget it. Layer after layer comes off and suddenly the student can be confronted by the fear that there will be nothing there when he gets to the centre of the onion. The Alexander Technique teaches us that there is something there at the centre, and that is the Flow which carries us physically, mentally and emotionally, and it is not something we can hold onto because it is fresh and spontaneous. The minute we try to fix it, it vanishes. When we trust it and flow with it we suddenly feel vitally alive and bubbly inside: no longer need we fear new situations, people or challenges because it is life challenging us to learn, grow and transform ourselves within the matrix of its being. We begin to grasp that there is no separation, there is not Life and us, there is only Life.

So many people are fixed, stuck at some particular stage of their evolutionary path. The whole of depth psychology and psychoanalysis has shown what damage is done when people carry unresolved emotional complexes which continue to influence their present situation and relationships. Certain changes, shocks and traumas were never properly processed and resolved. They were repressed and left scars of unconscious expectation which have influenced their lives ever since. People who are fixed inside are very often desperately looking for change to come from the outside in some way: a new partner to sweep them off their feet; winning the football pools; a lucky break in their business situation; a new job; emigrating... Whatever it is, the essential point is that the change, the rescue remedy, can only issue from within themselves, and until that inner transformation has been experienced their outer world will remain unchanged no matter how avidly they attempt to manipulate or change it from the outside. Gazing down at our reflection in a still pool, we may think that by beating the water with a stick we will manage to alter our reflection in some way, yet as soon as the water settles again we find our reflection unaltered, gazing back at us. Similar analogies abound, yet the point remains the same: we must transform from within if we would transform the world around us.

Those who understand the principles of self-transformation, and can work with them, discover that they hold in their hands the magic wand of purified perception which, alone, can transmute base metal into gold.

Chapter 8

PSYCHO-PHYSICAL REBALANCING

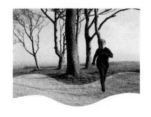

Ever since Alexander first discovered the principles of the Alexander Technique he always emphasised that his technique was a psycho-physical technique, that he was looking at the way that the mind and body interacted with each other. If you read *The Use of the Self,* which is the story of his discovery and how he made it, Alexander clearly describes how he was unable to solve the hoarseness in his voice or to release the muscular tension in his throat and neck muscles merely by physical self-manipulation or by trying to position himself in a different manner. He had to involve his thinking, or 'thought projections', in the attempt to change his habit patterns; and he also had to become aware of his own process, how he was straining and forcing himself in his effort to become the greatest actor the world had ever seen. He realised the futility of merely working on the physical level when attempting to change habit patterns, because man is a psycho-physical being - and, I would add, he is an emotional and spiritual being as well.

The problem with applying the Alexander Technique to a wider population has been that, whereas Alexander's system of directing energy flow within the body through 'directions' or maintaining thought projections is a system that is universally applicable to the whole population, his own particular process and the learning that he got from it is only particular to himself (and perhaps a few other people with very similar issues). For example, whereas Alexander discovered that he was a very ambitious personality with a tendency to force things, so much so that he was actually sabotaging his own efforts, another person might have the opposite problem, being completely passive, lacking in motivation and believing themselves to be a failure. So Alexander's process is not going to be of much significance to them. On the contrary they would have to learn how to develop their will-power more, to have faith and trust in themselves, and that it's OK for them to have needs and to have those needs fulfilled. Getting to a place where they can say, "I'm OK, and I deserve to have my needs met," would represent a significant step forward for them, one that brings more harmony and balance to their perspective.

Looking at these two opposite poles of the same problem it is interesting to see that they do have a similarity, in that they are linked by polarity and they both need to get back to a more balanced middle place. At that place the two opposite poles are integrated and there is an awareness of the whole range of possibilities, along the whole continuum; so that even though I might be at one particular point at this moment in time, I am also aware that I have experienced being at another place before, and that I am capable of shifting. Ultimately I might be able to say that I contain all polarities and all possibilities within myself, and that the way I am is now a matter of choice rather than a matter of compulsion. Or, to put it another way, I can be more detached about the place where I am at at this precise moment in time because I realise that it is essentially transitory - it will pass; it will change; I am not trapped in that particular way of being. Having this realisation, and understanding the mechanics of my personality structure better, I am also aware of what I need to do in order to get to another place - I can also use my will-power to change the way that I am. Because I've been to that other place before, I know what it feels like, that it's part of my potentiality.

Ultimately a one-line definition of the Alexander Technique might be that it is a way of changing habits. Not just physical habits but also mental and emotional ones, because habits go deep - they are a psycho-physical reality. Every thought that we think, every word that we utter, every emotional tremor that we feel, has a physical component as well. It is of inestimable value to learn how to decode that hidden body language. This was Alexander's discovery: that effective change is impossible without working on all these different levels.

Psychotherapists have also discovered this. Fritz Perls, the Father of Gestalt Psychotherapy, was influenced by the Alexander Technique in South Africa just after the Second World War. Although he didn't agree with Alexander's ideas about 'inhibition' and 'non-end-gaining' (because he was very much of the philosophy of getting needs met and achieving satisfaction at the end of the cycle without any inner or outer blockages interfering with the ability to complete), he was still impressed with the way that sensitivity to bodily sensations could be increased with the Alexander Technique. According to Fritz Perls you couldn't be in touch with your needs as a unique human being if you were not in touch with your bodily sensations, because sensation is the start of the cycle of awareness and needs satisfaction. He certainly agreed with Alexander's concept of 'faulty sensory appreciation', and how bad postural habits can cause us to partially or totally lose touch with what is actually happening in our bodies, because we accept a state of permanently over-tensed muscles as normal and as therefore not worth registering. Fritz Perls felt that we are out of touch with our emotions because we are out of touch with our bodies and are living too much in our heads. He would often make provocative overstatements such as 'lose your mind and come to your senses'.

Another eminent psychotherapist who also stressed the fact that we are psycho-physical organisms was Professor Eugene Gendlin of the University of Chicago. He was doing research into the question of why psychotherapy works with some people but not with others and what the differences between the two groups are. After researching into thousands of cases he found what he believed to be a causative factor, and using this he could even predict within the first few sessions who was going to benefit from therapy (and who was just going to waste their time and money). It was nothing to do with the therapist or even the method being used, it was simply an ability within the client to spot their own psycho-physical shifts at important points in their therapy, so that important insights did not just remain an intellectual insight but actually became a realisation of precisely what they were doing to themselves on a psycho-physical level, and what the options were so that the habit pattern could be altered.

In his book *Focusing* Professor Gendlin has outlined a simple six-step approach which shows people how they can activate this whole process on their own. In point of fact he specifically advocates that 'normal' people in the world, not just neurotics or severely damaged patients in therapy, should be able to learn this technique and use it as an essential life skill on a day-to-day basis. I would certainly agree with Professor Gendlin's ideas and it arouses the vision of a society in which a majority of people accept the view that life is a process of ongoing self-transformation. However, to contribute to this process effectively you have to have the skills and experience as well as the conviction that self-transformation is a practical necessity and a wonderful liberation at the same time.

We are at this time experiencing a period of major global, and also individual, transformation. Energy and awareness is on the increase, so this means that blockages and frustrations are intensified but at the same time the higher potentialities that we can contact to transform ourselves and raise our level of consciousness are also more accessible. So it becomes more and more unbearable just to stand still and be stuck in the same old rut, but also easier once you take the decision to move forward along the path of growth and change.

The question is *how to change effectively.* The force of habits goes deep; it is a physical, mental and emotional reality. You can recognise a bad habit yet still be powerless to change it. This is where the Paradoxical Theory of Change (Arnold Beissner) comes in. Briefly stated it is this: change occurs when one becomes what he is, not when he tries to become what he is not.

"Change does not take place through a coercive attempt by the individual or by another person to change him, but it does take place if one takes the time and effort to be what he is - to be fully invested in his current positions. By rejecting the role of change agent, we make meaningful and orderly change possible" (A. Beissner). This theory, which has played a large part in Gestalt Psychotherapy, at first seems totally paradoxical. It doesn't seem to make sense. My first reaction was: "So you're trying to tell me that if I desperately want and need to change, my best strategy is not to force anything but to just stay where I am and accept myself exactly as I am? How will that help? Come on, pull the other one!"

But if you start to think about it Paradoxical Psychology makes sense. Imagine that you have an eight-year-old child who doesn't want to eat her salad. You know that it's healthy to eat salad and that this little girl is not getting the vitamins that she needs from her diet. However the more you threaten and force her the more obstinate she becomes and the less likely she is to eat it. Coercion will not work, you have to be subtle. So try paradoxical psychology, and tell her, "Good, I'm really pleased that you don't want to eat your salad today. I love salad and there is more for me, yummy!" This is much more effective. That little girl is left there with a doubt at the back of her mind, "Maybe I'm missing out on something here. Maybe salad is really nice." After a few experiences like this the chances are that *she will ask you* for a portion of salad on her plate. It works because human nature is so paradoxical.

Now this theory has very interesting implications for the Alexander Technique and for giving directions. When we give directions we should always do so from a position of total self-acceptance. Even if there is an ache or pain behind that shoulder blade or in that knee, do not get into conflict with it and do not force it to change. That merely adds more tension (both mental and physical) to the situation and exacerbates it. Of course you do want it to change and to go away, but you have to be subtle about it. Paradoxical psychology is the way. For example, if you are standing and wish to give directions with the long-term objective to release muscular tension and to lengthen your spine you could say something like:

> *"I am aware of this distance from the top of my head*
> *down to my ankles and heels.*
> *I am this tall, and I do not need to be any taller,*
> *and I do not need to be any shorter,*
> *I accept myself totally as I am,*
> *I do not have to change because I am perfect already."*

You see the mind is a very tricky thing, you have to be subtle and trick your mind. After all, why shouldn't you? Because your mind is tricking you all the time with all those subconscious assumptions and expectations that are running your life, just below the level of conscious awareness. So paradoxical psychology is essential when giving directions, and it isn't even a game any more, because for that period of time whilst you are maintaining your directions and your thought projections it actually has to be 100 per cent real, absolutely convincing, for it to work, whilst you do not work, if you see what I mean.

Alexander obviously knew about these things instinctively, because his famous and original formulation of directions was :

> *"Let the neck be free,*
> *to let the head go forward and up,*
> *to let the back lengthen and widen."*

The original emphasis was on the word *let*, but human nature being what it is, beginners will tend to pick up on the words "go forward and up" and "lengthen and widen", which is completely counter-productive. We are all such doers that it takes a lot of self-observation in order to be able to spot that and turn it around, so that we learn the art of being, being more receptive, being a non-doer and letting things happen. Which is what Alexander's little word *let* is all about. Personally when I am teaching new students about the Alexander Technique I prefer to be very explicit and up-front about my precise meaning and not leave things to chance. Which is why I will be using some of my formulations of these directions rather than Alexander's.

I have called this aspect of the work 'psycho-physical rebalancing' because we all need to get back into balance, back to centre. An essential prerequisite for this is to develop that calm, relaxed awareness of ourselves in order to be open to our Inner Guidance.

Ordinarily our mind is agitated, our bodies tensed up, and our emotions too confused to be able to tune in with our Inner Intuitive Wisdom. First of all the breathing has to calm down, and then we can use the Alexander Technique in order to relax and realign the body. Then the mind has to become a calm instrument of awareness; we have to detach ourselves from our stream of thoughts and inner conflicts. Finally we have to reach a state of creative indifference about all of our emotional impulses, our likes and dislikes, our fears and compulsions. Obviously this is easier said than done, which is why we need psycho-physical rebalancing on a daily basis, in order to process our stuff and get back into harmony and balance again. The mind can rationalise anything, and it is doing that most of the time. The body cannot lie, which is why I find it an indispensable instrument for getting to the truth of the situation.

What we have to remember is that the body thinks. It's a slower sort of thinking than is going on in our mind, but it still thinks. And it is a deeper level of thought and awareness. In general I find that I can have about 20 ordinary fleeting thoughts in the time that it takes me to fully register one body sensation. So this is automatically taking the brain into alpha rhythms, the state associated with meditation and deep inspirational thought, as opposed to beta rhythms, which is more our everyday state of cognitive awareness and quick mental associations. In alpha rhythms we are more capable of contacting our intuition and the guidance of our higher spiritual self, and we have the calmness and the receptivity to do so.

Now if you believe, as I do, that we are one whole, complete, psycho-physical organism then it follows that we will be receptive to our spiritual help and guidance all over. Parts of our body will start to resonate when we are attuned. We will start to register shifts in our bodies, in our musculature and joints, that are signals as to the direction of our growth and unfolding. We all carry a muscular memory in our bodies of our shocks and traumas, of our fears and tensions. If there is to be real growth and change it has to be a whole psycho-physical shift, not just a cognitive insight whilst we remain locked in the prison house of our psycho-physical habit patterns. So it makes complete sense that when we are receiving guidance from our Higher Self, that it will be psycho-physical guidance, subtle shifts and releases within the tension patterns of our musculature, combined with cognitive insights that are pointing the way forward for our future unfolding. There is no hidden agenda of the teacher here. Each student works through their issues at their own pace and time, but we become much more detached and aware of the learning experience behind each issue that we are facing, and we can receive the subtle promptings of our Higher Spiritual Self that is pointing the way forwards.

It actually doesn't matter what your particular concept of your Higher Self is, or even if you are totally agnostic and don't have one - what is important is following the principles. The three steps of self-transformation work.

(1) Be aware of what the problem is, admit it, name it.

(2) Admit that you cannot solve it in your present state; so either surrender it to your Inner Intuitive Guidance, just open yourself and be receptive to that guidance; or else just empty yourself, admit that you are 'at the end of your tether', that you cannot go any further by your own efforts and admit that you have reached a state of total self-surrender. This is actually the best place to be when dealing with major problems and crises.

Do not be frightened at this point; stay with that sense of futility or helplessness and hopelessness - the desert is about to become fertile in a most miraculous manner. The principle is the same, all religions teach it, empty yourself, create a vacuum and God will be sucked in - irrespective of whether you believe in Him or not.

(3) An answer begins to emerge in the dark mysterious womb of space. At first rather nebulous and indistinct. Be sensitive and prepared to follow your subtle inner psycho-physical shifts, your intuitive feelings, the voice of your conscience, your 'hunches' or however your inner intuitive guidance works. These are small tender shoots and need to be nurtured and protected from the huge trampling monsters of doubt, neglect and disbelief. Be attentive, watch without forcing it, have focused awareness without tension, reach a state of creative indifference.

Because the Alexander Technique is a psycho-physical technique, when I work with students the answer generally emerges as a felt bodily sense. This is not the only way that it can be felt, because the voice of intuition can speak in many ways, but the essential prerequisite is a deep inner calmness which means that all the muscles have to be relaxed and you have to reach this state of creative indifference - which is deep mental and emotional calmness. The bodily felt intuition is the most reliable because it is the most truthful; the mind alone is a very tricky instrument that is capable of misleading us with its hidden agendas. The famous Swiss psychologist Dr CG Jung, speaking of the benefits of yoga, wrote: "Yoga practice ... would be ineffectual without the concepts on which yoga is based. It combines the bodily and the spiritual in an extraordinarily complete way. In the East, where these ideas and practices have developed, and where for several thousand years an unbroken tradition has created the necessary spiritual foundations, yoga is, as I can readily believe, the perfect and appropriate method of fusing body and mind together so that they form a unity which is scarcely to be questioned. This unity creates a psychological disposition which makes possible intuitions that transcend consciousness." Many people have remarked that the Alexander Technique is a western form of yoga, that recognises the psycho-physical unity of man and that seeks to integrate this awareness into everyday activities. From this basis of calmness, openness and receptivity we have laid the foundation for a reliable intuition, and an effective inner spiritual guidance and direction of our lives.

These intuitions are very fleeting, they are small tender shoots that are easily forgotten - significantly enough, because we all have a huge vested interest in staying where we are and not changing, because life is so frightening that it feels safer to stay put with the devil you know, even if it is a very uncomfortable, constricting place being locked up with that old devil in that demoralising, familiar space. The devil's argument is always, "Don't be stupid; how do you know that there is anything better out there? It's a dangerous world; it hasn't treated you well up till now, has it? So why expect anything better? Stay where you are." This is a very insidious argument that isn't even rational, but it is powerful, emotional and fearful. However, the other main reason we stay put is because these defences were at one time our best way of coping with a very difficult situation; they were our way of surviving in terrifying situations, and the memory of that is stored in the subconscious mind and is locked into the tension patterns of the body.

These negative expectations are very hard to shift. In traditional psychotherapy *probably the major role of the psychotherapist is to give the client a completely different experience of what the 'other person' can be like in a relationship,* in an honest dialogue, despite the counter-transference and the subtle, covert manipulation of the client to get the therapist to repeat their experiences and materialise their expectations of how they deserve to be treated in life by others. This is probably the most significant learning of the therapeutic relationship; of how our expectations have created our reality, and the experience of how things can be different and better. This can take years of patient learning and it is the experience of this rather than what is actually said in therapy that counts.

In psycho-physical work we are not concerned with the content of a client's story so much as the process of what is happening in the whole psycho-physical organism. So we don't have endless rounds of discussing, for example, how the client got involved in this abusive relationship, what went on and how they eventually left amidst tears and recriminations. Yes, it is important to hear the story, but then the question is not so much what happened as *how it is happening, right now* as they are recounting this story and thinking about this relationship. What muscles are tensing? What contortions are occurring in their body posture? What is happening to their breathing? As they get into this particular posture, this pattern of holding, what does it feel like emotionally? For example, the client might be feeling sad after their partner left, the chest feels heavy and constricted, particularly around the heart, s/he gets an image of a hand clutching a heart, "It feels like I'm being squeezed dry." OK, we have an image to work with, a statement from their body wisdom. How does this resonate with their life situation? Instead of playing victim and saying, "I'm being squeezed dry," can they change it around, take responsibility, take ownership and say, *"I am squeezing myself dry"*? That is a completely different perspective, isn't it? If it had a voice what would this hand say? These are all classical Gestalt interventions, and are very powerful in their own right. They open the work up, setting the stage for some sort of experiment; perhaps some sort of enactment or dramatisation will follow. That is fine. However, the psycho-physical therapist who is also a trained Alexander Technique teacher has another possibility: direct, hands-on work that is very powerful and opens up all sorts of interesting implications.

Through using the Technique we can project directions along the length of the spine and out through the top of the head, whilst keeping the body still and all the muscles perfectly relaxed around the central axis of the spinal column. The question that is then posed to the client's Body Wisdom is this: "Body Wisdom, you have a memory of what it was like when everything was perfect - what would it feel like if everything were to come back to balance and harmony on the physical, mental, emotional and spiritual levels?" And both therapist and client remain perfectly still and wait for the Inner Intuitive Guidance, working through the body process by a series of very subtle bodily shifts, to point the way forwards.

I'll give a few examples. One client had chronic neck and jaw tension as a result of whiplash after a serious car crash. He said that his jaw felt like an iron plate bolted back into his neck, and the sides of his neck felt like lots of stretched rubber bands pulling down the sides of his neck and into his shoulders. We worked on these patterns using directions and the Alexander Technique. As the tension patterns in his neck and jaw released (for the first time in months!) and as we walked around the room I asked him how he felt different now. He came up with the words:

"My heels are drilling down through the floorboards
and into the ground,
I am solid, I am stable,
My jaw is soft and smooth. My neck is fat and chunky."

These are his words that he had come up with from his own Body Wisdom. So I told him, "That's your affirmation for the week. Use it when you want to get back into this space again and dispel the traumatic memory of your accident." It was quite a breakthrough for someone who had been in agony for the last few months. What is also significant is that, for someone with severe neck and shoulder tensions, any release can only take place in relationship to what is happening in the pelvis and legs, so part of his body process was to learn how to trust the earth again, to get more grounded and to release his weight into the earth through his heels.

Another client felt 'put down' by her boss at work. This resulted in shoulder tension which she experienced as a metal brace across the top of her shoulders with round caps around her shoulder joints. The joints felt mummified, and she also felt as if she shouldn't smile at people for fear of antagonising her supervisor. The message that she was getting was, "You are unimportant here, don't spend so much time socialising." We worked with the Alexander Technique and giving directions and a whole pattern of release began to spread throughout her body as her back began to lengthen and widen and the tension left her shoulders and neck muscles. This was beautiful for her to experience but the really important question was how to pinpoint with words how she felt different about herself on the mental and emotional levels as well. She came up with the words:

> *"I'm free,*
> *I'm happy,*
> *I'm a whole person."*

I said, "That's fine, that's it, that's your affirmation for the week. Work with it every day, especially when your supervisor gets dangerously close to you and you feel yourself tensing up in the shoulders again in response to all those unspoken or spoken messages. He is trying to put you down; you don't have to put yourself down even further by tensing your shoulders and neck and facial muscles.

"Repeat the affirmation and then pause for a second or two to feel the resonance in your body. Wait for the echo. These are powerful words, chosen by your own body wisdom. These words will trigger off an actual physiological response pattern in your body. So, just pause for a minute now, and take a mental snapshot of how you feel in your totality right now. Store that away in your muscular memory, so that when you say these words again, it's going to trigger off the total psycho-physical response pattern. These aren't just words, I want you to actually feel the physical changes within yourself as the shoulder muscles lengthen and release, as the neck muscles free up and the facial muscles soften and become more responsive again.

"These physiological changes will actually act as a source of support within you; you will feel different about yourself; the words will ring true because they are supported by your own inner, physical experience of yourself as being different. Because your body language is now different you will find that people, and your supervisor in particular, will react to you differently next week. It's an unspoken thing; it's direct communication through body language, it's direct communication to the subconscious mind."

Modern scientific research is opening up a new field, it is called *psychoneuroimmunology.* This is producing solid scientific evidence to show how a patient's state of mind and emotions will affect their immune system - that is, their ability to fight off diseases and stay healthy. But it isn't just the immune system that can be affected by our thoughts and feelings: it is the glands of the endocrine system; it is the neurological system and the gastrointestinal system as well. This is an information flow that links all the different systems across the body, and this actually represents a second, chemical-based nervous system. Briefly, what happens is that *ligands* (which can be thought of as information molecules) lock onto *receptors* in cell walls and transmit information that changes the way that that cell works. There are *neurotransmitters* that are produced in the brain to carry information across the gap, or synapse, between one neuron and the next in the brain. Then there are *steroids* which include the sex hormones, and finally the largest group of all which is *peptides* which float through the fluids of the body, the bloodstream and the cerebrospinal fluid, and play a wide role in regulating practically all life processes. These ligands travel long distances causing complex and fundamental changes in the cells whose receptors they lock onto.

There is not space to go into greater detail here; anyone who wants to find out more about this can read Candace Pert's excellent book *"The Molecules of Emotion". The interesting and fundamental point however is that prolonged emotional trauma or stress can affect the production of these chemicals, thus throwing the whole system out of balance and retaining a memory of the trauma at the deepest cellular level.* This is one of the fascinating conclusions of the latest scientific research in this field. Of course the drug companies are in there saying, "Well, your illness is due to too much of this, or too little of that so take our drugs and we will correct the chemical imbalance for you." But this is still only treating the symptom and not the cause. True healing can only take place through a psycho-physical therapy form that unlocks the memory of the original trauma, allows a resolution of that problem from a new and higher perspective (your intuitive body wisdom), and then generates a positive mental affirmation that can keep alive the reality of that new psycho-physical release.

An interesting piece of scientific research has been done to prove this point in an experiment with baby monkeys. A group of baby monkeys were given enough bottled milk for their needs but were deprived of physical touch, love and cuddles. Pretty soon they all showed signs of trauma and depression, which is to be expected. This affected the hypothalamus which is part of the limbic system or the emotional brain. This caused increased levels of a neuropeptide called CRF (cortical releasing factor) which, when it hit the pituitary gland, stimulated the secretion of the peptide ACTH, which then travels through the bloodstream to the adrenal glands where it binds to specific receptors on the adrenal cell walls. The adrenal glands, as we know, control the production of adrenalin, which causes the fight-or-flight alarm response, which helps us to deal with conditions of extreme danger.

However, another thing that the adrenal glands do is to produce the steroid corticosterone, which is necessary for healing and damage control when an injury has occurred. These steroids are very stress-inducing. Imagine these baby monkeys (and human beings in a similar situation) having greatly increased levels of this steroid, corticosterone, pumping around their bloodstream saying something like, "There is an emergency here; you are about to be damaged; you are about to be hurt but we are prepared to deal with damage as and when it occurs." This continues for days and weeks and possibly even months.

Because we are a psycho-physical unity, and there is this feedback loop, these are the sorts of thoughts and emotions that we will get from having large quantities of this steroid in the bloodstream. Your expectation is that you are about to get hurt; you might well say that these are the steroids of negative expectations. So there is not only an initial trauma, but the memory of that trauma is retained in the body over time. The memory of trauma is retained in the high levels of the neuropeptide CRF (which is 10 times higher than normal in suicide cases) and the high steroid levels in the bloodstream; it is retained in the production of the hypothalamus, the pituitary and the adrenal glands; it is retained in the very cells of the body. This body memory persists over time and, due to the psycho-physical feedback loop, it will affect people's thoughts and expectations. So production levels of CRF and the steroids will not go down. It sounds like the same sort of habitual closed-circle that Alexander had to deal with when he was giving his Shakespearean recitals on stage, except now modern science has explained how it takes place in the glands, the fluids, the very cells of our bodies.

Anyway, to get back to these baby monkeys who were the subjects of this cruel experiment. They were depressed and stressed at the same time, and there was a disrupted feedback loop that failed to signal that CRF levels were getting too high. Then they brought on the 'monkey hug therapist', an older monkey who constantly hugged and cuddled the stressed-out baby monkeys. Within a short period of time they were cured and all the chemical symptoms were reversed. The hugging broke the feedback loop sending the message, "We don't need any more steroids because the trauma is over, we feel fine." The high CRF levels came down. This shows the value of physical contact in therapy and also that if the positive reparative message can be repeated consistently over a period of time the damage can be reversed on a chemical and a cellular level.

This is my argument for psycho-physical rebalancing and positive affirmations that reaffirm not only the new mental insight *but also the physical sensation of that new positive space.* These are, I believe, changing the body memory of the trauma and affecting the cellular feedback loop. Therapy is fine for a while, and so are support groups where you can go to get hugs, physical contact and support. But it must not become an addiction or a way of life. There comes a time when you have to be able to find a way to process your own emotional traumas, and to find an inner strength and security from within. Psycho-physical rebalancing, which is based on the principles of the Alexander Technique, provides an inner connection to the support and guidance of your Body Wisdom. Thus you can ground yourself in a newly rebalanced physical, mental and emotional reality. This is a way of breaking habit patterns. This is a way of influencing the feedback loop of that second chemical nervous system.

UNLOCKING THE CIRCLE - UNLEASHING THE SPIRAL

Every thought that we think, every word that we utter, and every emotional tremor that we feel has a physical resonance. Thus oft-repeated thoughts or an extremely traumatic emotional experience can become a part of our body memory and manifest as physical tension patterns in the body.

We often get locked into a vicious circle, where certain thoughts and emotions cause a particular physical tension pattern, and conversely just being in that particular posture causes us to think and feel in a certain way. It is very difficult to break out of a closed circle like this; without outside help it is often impossible. We have to be able to introduce a circuit breaker at some point, either psychologically or physically, in order to break out of the groove and show that some sort of change is possible. Actually, in all of my psycho-physical work I have found that the key breakthrough always comes when the client is able *to take responsibility for their reaction pattern, for their part in perpetuating the drama.* It is easy to blame the past and to blame other people, but that keeps you in a disempowered place in the role of victim. It is only when you can take responsibility for your own thoughts and actions, including your body language and state of consciousness, that you can give out different messages to the world and get a different response.

CASE STUDY JOHN: **lack of achievement in life**

(Names and details in this case study have been changed in order to preserve client confidentiality).

One client John came to me with issues around lack of self worth, under-achievement and bad posture. He knew the type of psycho-physical work that I did, and that it would be necessary to work with understanding and transforming the physical *and* emotional blockages before he could mobilise more energy and achieve his goals in life. So I asked him to focus on his physical sensations first of all and then to see what thoughts or images or emotions came up for him that linked to these sensations. The most immediate sensations he noticed was that his head felt hazy and spaced out. He felt a lack of energy in his body and a lack of mental focus. He felt disconnected both from himself and from the world. It was a familiar space to him, because he seemed to have been there for most of his life. "It's like *floating in limbo*".....he said. The words of a well known song came floating through his mind .... "I have become comfortably numb......"

I asked him "what do these words and physical sensations link to? What does this mean in the story of your life, if you look at the whole film of your life, does this make any sense to you at all?" A picture of his mother appeared on the inner screen of his consciousness. (Well if it's not one thing its your mother!). I asked him "why is she still so powerful after all of these years?" He answered: "she made me feel impotent, put the fear of God into me about sex being dirty and wicked so that I was scared stiff of making any sexual advances to girls, and all my sexual drive remained locked up inside me as sexual fantasies. Not being allowed to connect my passion to my life, no wonder I feel disconnected to myself."

I challenged him: "Your mother might well have been responsible for starting this pattern of behaviour in you, but she isn't around now. Rather than heaping all the blame on figures from the dim and distant past (which is another way of keeping yourself impotent), is there any way that you can take ownership of your behaviour in *the present moment* that keeps you disempowered?"

John thought awhile, then he answered simply: "by not allowing myself to feel alive and not going with my enthusiasm........... This feeling of a lack of energy in my body is beginning to make sense. If I don't allow myself to flow with my enthusiasm then it is hard to be motivated in life. It all becomes so boring. If it's dangerous and forbidden to have sexual thoughts then it's also dangerous to tolerate a high energy charge in the body *about anything,* because I associate that with sexuality. I don't allow myself to want anything with a powerful enough energy charge to make it happen".

He sighed and thought for a while. "I remember when I was little and wanted a bicycle. I was 12 at the time and I wanted so much to get that latest model racing bike - but I wasn't allowed to have it, I was told that there wasn't enough money, squashed into not wanting it any more, into shutting up which is the same thing as shutting down. So I made the decision *not* to want and not to ask for things anymore, it was easier. But it left me with this feeling of being disconnected from myself and from the world, of being disempowered". I asked John where he felt that feeling of disconnection through excessive muscular tension most acutely. He explored his physical sensations for a while and then answered: "in the pelvic region".

Having defined the problem I knew that it was now time to work with John on the table, using the Psycho-Physical Rebalancing Technique that I have described earlier in this chapter. Having worked for so many years in this way I knew that the wisdom and guidance of his own "Body Wisdom" would be able to restore perfect peace and harmony on all levels, and to point out the way forwards. I asked him to give directions along the spine and out through the crown of his head, bringing his mind back to the crown of his head every time his attention wandered. Going with the flow we entered a timeless, spaceless zone; as John attained a state of calmness and interiorisation his energies began to flow freely and subtle bodily shifts began to take place. His inner self began to open, and John's consciousness clarified itself. I asked him to focus his attention on the bodily shifts that had taken place and what they meant for him. Eventually he came up with these words:

My heart is free

I'm feeling bubbly and alive
My arms and shoulders are full of energy

I feel solid and grounded in my pelvis
I feel connected to all of myself

I am a child of the universe
All good can come to me

I wrote down these words for John so that he had something to take away with him and use whenever the old fears started to recur. These words might not mean very much to another person, nor would they be particularly effective, but for John they became powerful trigger words, transformative sounds of great potency. I explained that the way to use a personal affirmation is to repeat and then pause for a few seconds, repeat and then pause. It is in the few seconds of silence that the words filter down and strongly resonate in the muscles, joints, and sinews, recreating through the power of association, the positive pattern of release that he had felt during our table work together. Thus John now had a powerful tool that could enable him to break out of his vicious negative cycle into an upward spiral of positive physical sensations, thoughts, and feelings.

Body Wisdom is innate to each and every person. It is not imposed from without by a teacher, or by theoretical models. This Wisdom seeks to lead us toward our highest good through our psycho-physical intuitions. These tender shoots deserve recognition and careful nurturing if we are to grow and transform ourselves into our full potential. It is not enough just to have a good insight and then forget it. It takes time and effort to practise it, often under challenging conditions, to repeat it until it becomes a reliable part of our psycho-physical being and to integrate it in our lives. Only then have we truly transformed ourselves on all levels. This is the power of the positive affirmations generated by our Body Wisdom.

Chapter 9

ATTAINING PSYCHOLOGICAL BALANCE

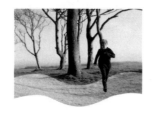

S tress is the curse of our times. Many people seem to be busy, busy, much too busy. Too busy to talk, too busy to relate, too busy to be in touch with themselves. It is as if time has shrunk and there are only 20 hours to the day now instead of the 24 hours there used to be. There is a constant sense of speed and restless activity that results in an increased heart rate, increased blood pressure, shortness of breath and unnecessary muscular tension - and that is just the background tension pattern! Stress rates zoom upwards in psychologically demanding situations, for example, when giving a presentation or a performance, in a job interview, being criticised at work, making important decisions, trying to meet a deadline. Each time there is extra stress the psychological and physiological tension increases even more.

The Alexander Technique can provide an invaluable tool for dealing capably with psychologically demanding situations. It provides an inner base, an inner sense of solidity and calmness that acts like an anchor and stops you shooting up into your head, into the realm of panic and disconnected thoughts. In the previous chapter on psycho-physical rebalancing a process was outlined, based on the Alexander Technique, of opening up the inner energy flow so that you can process your own individual meaning that lies behind a stressful reaction pattern. What is it in your life history that has contributed to the way you are now in this situation? How are you helping to recreate that situation in the present moment? How can you create a new, more balanced pattern for the future? This will help you to deal with the deeper underlying issues and to deal with your past conditioning - which is absolutely crucial. However, when you are right in the middle of a stressful situation you need something immediate that is going to help you to relax physically and stay focused mentally. That is exactly what the Alexander Technique can do for you.

Suppose you are a businessman facing a deadline on a deal, or a housewife trying to get the house cleaned, or a student trying to get an essay in on time - there is a lot to be done and seemingly very little time to do it in. Anyone facing any sort of deadline is under pressure and this can be very stress-inducing. The natural tendency of the mind is to start going through your 'things to do list' - I'm doing 'a', but I still have 'x', 'y' and 'z' to do and I'll never manage it on time! The mind starts panicking, the muscles start tensing, the heartbeat, respiration rate and blood pressure all increase, and the end result is that you are even less capable of focusing your mind and energies on the job at hand. Effective time management is based on two things:

(1) strategic planning so that you are aware of what your long-term objectives are and what the top priority is right now that you need to focus on, and

(2) creating a time slot in which you focus on that top priority efficiently.

Rather than thinking repeatedly, "I've got to get this finished, but time is running out," and feeling tense and breathless, create a timeless zone by erecting mental barriers that will keep out the approach of encroaching worries, like 'x', 'y' and 'z', that cloud the mind. Through the strength of your mind, of your thought projections, which has now been trained through the practice of giving 'directions', it is possible to create a worry-free zone of time in which you can now give full attention to a top priority project. Mentally, you can say to yourself, for example, "OK, from nine till

12 noon I've got three hours to focus on this project; this is an oasis of time, quality time to give my full attention to this subject and to produce quality work. Whatever is produced within this three-hour time slot is fine. I don't have to complete, I just have to stay mentally focused, physically relaxed and let my thoughts flow freely." How enjoyable it now seems, three whole hours to stay within the boundaries of this worry-free zone creating beautiful work, what fun! Just with a simple shift of attitude like this it is amazing how you can create mental relaxation instead of stress, and the paradox is of course that when the pressure is off and the inner creativity is freed up you are much more likely to produce quality work.

This is of course a circular process, because stress is a psycho-physical phenomenon. So giving 'directions' to *allow* the neck to be free, to *let* the jaw release forwards and the head release upwards, to *let* the back lengthen and widen, so that you are sitting firmly grounded in your pelvis feeling light and supported from the ground up, breathing easily - this all adds to a feeling of solidity, calmness and mental focus. By reducing physical tension you do feel calmer, less stressed and able to think more clearly. Even when you are under intense pressure, say the report really does need to be handed in by 12 noon today, the same principles still apply. Calm yourself down using the Alexander Technique and instead of getting totally panicked you can occasionally affirm:

"Everything will be done perfectly in the time available."

It takes the same amount of time and energy to keep repeating this positive affirmation to yourself as it does to be thinking stressful and negative thoughts. Believe it or not, the power of the mind is such that you do actually complete the task, against all odds, exactly to the minute.

Another psychologically challenging situation is being interviewed for a job. The Alexander Technique can help you to improve your communication skills when being interviewed by calming you down and allowing you to understand what you are communicating through your body language. Realise that the worst thing that can happen is that you may not be offered the job. But do you really want it, anyway? What are the disadvantages? What do *you* think of the firm and the person who is interviewing you? You need to shift your mental attitude in order to preserve your sense of self-worth and to get to a more balanced place. Above all pause ('inhibit') and don't rush into any decisions. It is always best to sleep on it before coming to a final conclusion in order to give your intuition time to work.

Conversely, when you are the interviewer the Alexander Technique improves your interviewing skills by teaching you to read another person's body language. It helps you to spot any inner conflicts or lack of clarity during negotiations, highlights any incongruity between the verbal and non-verbal messages, and improves listening skills by teaching a more open, sympathetic body language. As 70 per cent of our communication is non-verbal, observing and understanding another person's body language - their facial expression, tone of voice, gesture and posture - are essential. These are all vital clues that help to reveal a person's feeling state, which may be different from their verbal communications. Often this communication is subconscious and part of a vague 'total impression' of a person, but you can make this understanding specific and accurate. What exactly can you hear in a voice, see in a posture or read into a gesture or facial expression? Through the practice of the Alexander Technique you will find that you develop a very accurate understanding of other people's body language by letting it resonate in your own body and feelings. You will develop your practical skills in reading other people's body language.

Many people can find it stressful to be criticised at work, or at home. There may be a psycho-physical issue going back to childhood that causes them to either feel small and annihilated when criticised by an authority figure or their partner, or else there may be a major reaction to an apparently trivial criticism as they explode with uncontrollable rage. Neither reaction is healthy. The individual story needs to be looked at using the technique of psycho-physical rebalancing, but the outline of the drama remains the same. The adult is all-powerful and all-knowing, and therefore when a mistake has been made the child is made to feel guilty and powerless. Therefore, when you recreate your childhood dramas with others in later life, when you are criticised, that particular button is pressed and you make the other person who is criticising you into an authority figure that is all-powerful, all-knowing and in the right! The little child inside you feels annihilated again, and no wonder you feel powerless to defend yourself or else explode in a rage that is in direct proportion to the inner feelings of impotence.

The recent research of Alan Shor has shown that our memory is not just mental, it is also emotional and somatic, remembered simultaneously in both the left and right hemispheres in different and simultaneous processes. For example, a frowning, critical face leads to fear and anxiety and the sensation of the stomach churning all at the same time. The psycho-physical memory from childhood is being recreated. If all that is triggered off by criticism by your boss or your partner at home then it needs looking at through psycho-physical rebalancing.

To achieve psychological balance it is very important to connect with your adult 'I' in the present moment (what do I want? ...I think? ...I need? etc.). To do this you have to be able to use a technique, like the Alexander Technique, that will help you to create your own space and time so that you can contact your pelvis and find out what you really want and need from that deep level of your being. But to do that you have to be able to disconnect from your fear, your guilt and your projection of omnipotence and omniscience onto the other (all of which is causing you to tense, especially in your lower back) and to see the other person as also having faults, processes and projections as well, and to negotiate (adult to adult) with that other, less-than-perfect being. At the same time you have to be big enough to admit it if you have made a mistake. That phraseology says it all, doesn't it? *To be big enough to admit that you have made a mistake.* You actually need to have a physical sensation of solidity and spaciousness, especially within the pelvis and the lower back, that is large enough to contain an admission of fault without being overwhelmed by it. "Yes, I have made a mistake for which I apologise and it won't happen again." (But that is only a small part of me the rest of me is OK I can still maintain my feelings of self-respect and pride for who I am and everything that I stand for.) In this way your breathing and nervous system are calmed down, you retain your mental focus and awareness and you don't block your energy flow.

Maintaining a sense of inner space and calm is also crucial in problem-solving. In the same way that people allow themselves to become overwhelmed by the pressure of time and deadlines, they can also become overwhelmed by the pressure of problems that need solving. Many people live in hope of a problem-free existence in some utopia, but problems are a part of life and *it is the way in which you solve your problems* that determines the quality your life, not the number of problems waiting to be solved. Do you see yourself as bigger than your problems, or do you see your problems as bigger than you? This is a crucial difference and one that can be shifted with the help of the Alexander Technique. When you see the problem as bigger than you, you go into stress and panic mode and you can feel overwhelmed and powerless. In a very real sense *you are recreating* your earlier life experience of feeling incompetent and powerless, because you are actually totally incapable of solving a problem in this mode. There are always several options available and one of them is the perfect solution to that particular problem, but you just cannot see it if you feel stressed out, or helpless and hopeless - your mind just isn't calm enough to work clearly in that situation. The Alexander Technique can change all of that.

The first step is to calm down and do nothing at all - it is always better to do nothing rather than rush in, do the wrong thing and make the problem worse. The next step is to give 'directions' to:

> "*allow* the neck to be free,
>   to *let* the jaw release forwards and the head upwards,
>   to *let* the back lengthen and widen."

Especially work on the 'directions' to *allow* the back to lengthen down from the hollow at the back of your neck, down to the coccyx at the base of the spine. When you feel that you have touched base so that the bottom of your pelvis is properly grounded and solid, give 'directions' to *allow* a widening across the back of your pelvis. When this starts working it gives a great sense of stability, because it is an upside down 'T'-joint and this will allow a sense of lengthening and release along the length of the spine. Now *allow* the stomach muscles to release and *allow* the breath to come in by itself (but slightly assist the out-breath to empty the lungs completely). As the breathing calms down the front side of the pelvis also releases so that there is a sense of space in the whole pelvic girdle. This induces a feeling of solidity and calmness and, as we are psycho-physical beings, this starts to allow the mind to work smoothly and calmly.

Once your mind is working clearly you can start calmly looking at all the existing options and brainstorming for new ones. Most importantly there is a release and expansion throughout the whole volume of the body, so that you are now big enough physically and psychologically to *contain* the problem within yourself. If you use the Alexander Technique in this way and keep calmly thinking about even the largest problems it is amazing how things gradually become clearer until a workable solution appears and the problem finally disappears. Even if there appears to be nothing that can be done, it is still possible to mentally contain the problem within the boundaries of your larger self. Say to yourself, "This is just a problem to be dealt with and I am bigger than this. There is nothing I can do at the moment, but while there's life there's hope, and I'm giving the problem over to my subconscious mind to deal with while I get on with other, more productive, work." With this attitude you will be surprised how the perfect solution will emerge with time.

It is the same with decision-making. Some people are paralysed with fear when they have to make an important, life-changing decision. They are simply unable to decide one way or another and so they procrastinate and nothing gets done. Others are unsure of what to do and allow themselves to get pushed into a decision by other stronger-willed people. The result is disastrous because a rushed decision is never a good decision, and if all the implications haven't been thought through fully you are pretty likely to want to change your mind as soon as the picture becomes clearer. The Alexander Technique can help you to develop clarity provided you give yourself enough time to *allow* the perfect decision to emerge. The key to it all is to pause ('inhibit') and don't rush into anything that you are not sure about. Take out a piece of paper and write a list of all the pros and cons for option one. Then on a separate piece of paper write out all the pros and cons for option two. Perhaps there is even an option three or four and you need to do the same thing for these options. To take a concrete example, suppose I were thinking of a career change in midlife and becoming a teacher, I might sit down and write something like the following:

OPTION ONE - Become a Teacher

Pros

1. Regular income
2. Get a pension
3. Long holidays
4. Worthwhile profession
5. Give something back to the community
6. Could work part-time
7. Build a raport with the younger generation

Cons

1. Have to maintain discipline
2. Could lose my temper quite often
3. Stressful job
4. Long hours preparing and marking schoolwork during term time
5. Working according to a central curriculum
6. No part in the decision-making process
7. Lack of spirituality in the school system
8. I have to do a year's conversion training on a student grant
9. I enjoy what I'm doing already

This is a carefully thought out list of the pros and cons (which many thoughtful people might do in this situation). But there is still no way of telling what separate weighting should be allocated to each item, which would then determine the overall balance of the decision. Having done everything possible to reach a rational decision, it is now time to ask your body wisdom and your higher intuitive faculty. Placing both hands palms downwards on this piece of paper I give 'directions' to *allow* a state of clear energy flow, I empty my mind completely of all preconceptions so that I reach a state of 'creative indifference' as to the outcome. I then wait to see how my body reacts on a holistic level. The back of my neck tenses, I feel as if I am carrying a heavy burden and my posture starts to crumple, I feel stressed and breathless. The answer is clearly a "No" because the body feeling has been so negative, and when I now look at the list in the Cons column it is obvious that items 1, 3 and 4 are very significant disadvantages for me and far outweigh anything in the Pros column. I can look at the whole decision quite clearly now and luckily I have been saved from becoming a teacher in the state educational system. Actually, on balance, I think I am much better suited to remain as a teacher of the Alexander Technique. When the decision is positive the bodily intuitions are very positive, expansive, light and joyous. Which is the complete opposite of the case here. As you gain experience in this method you will learn to trust it more and more.

This method is invaluable in helping to gain clarity in life because it utilises both the logical and the intuitive sides of the brain simultaneously. Relying solely on intuition can be disastrous, just as trusting to logic alone can be misleading, because you do not know how to weight the different factors. Using both together leads to clarity. Everything in life rests on clarity and the power of decision. Actually the whole secret of a successful life is being clear about what you want and then being prepared to wait long enough until you get exactly that, and not to settle for inferior substitutes beforehand. Which, if you think about it, is just another application of the law of 'direction' and 'inhibition'.

In the business world, giving presentations can be very stress-inducing for some people. Apart from the obvious problem of content, how to organise the material into some sort of coherent whole and how to present your key concepts in a powerful and memorable way, there are the inner issues: how to silence the inner critic; freedom from fear when presenting; maintaining self-confidence under pressure; improving your voice projection and how to connect with your enthusiasm and make an impact on your audience.

The inner critic can be completely destructive. It will say things like, "This stinks", "I am no good", "I wonder what all those people are thinking about me", "I look terrible", "I sound terrible", "Am I making any sense at all today?", "Why is everyone having such a negative reaction to me?", "I'm mucking it up again." Everyone has these negative tapes that can play through their heads at unwanted moments. These are either based on past conditioning or are prompted by fear. If they are based on past conditioning then it is important to deal with the deep, underlying issues through using psycho-physical rebalancing (as outlined in the previous chapter) so that your life is no longer being controlled by subconscious motivations. If it is a fearful reaction based in the moment then you need to use the principles of the Alexander Technique in order to become grounded, calm the breathing, get your directions flowing and get your mind working smoothly and calmly once again.

I can remember when I was first asked to give a presentation in front of a group. I just went into blind panic. I noticed I was taking short shallow breaths, and being out of breath affected my voice projection and my mental focus. My knees were shaking and my hands were sweating. I shot off at great speed speaking much too fast, and pretty soon I noticed that my audience had lost interest and most people had switched off. This reinforced all my negative tapes, which kept intruding into my thinking. I lost confidence completely, my posture collapsed, my voice dropped and I finished on a lame, apologetic note. A wonderful example of how not to give a presentation!

At my next attempt I tried being better prepared with small cue cards and dressing more smartly. But it still only improved matters slightly. I still had a horrible lump at the back of my throat, my voice was pinched and I was unable to feel at ease with myself or my audience. So after that I decided to use what I had learnt from the Alexander Technique. While I was just waiting my turn to speak, what I noticed in particular was how ungrounded I was and how tense my throat was. So I worked on my breathing, making sure that I completely emptied my lungs before *allowing* the air to flow back in by itself, giving it time to fill the lungs without forcing it. This calmed things down slightly. Then I worked on giving general directions to, *Allow the neck to be free.* Maintaining a thought projection along the length of the neck, so that I was observing the length without trying to make it longer or shorter, was of particular benefit in calming down the panic reaction. It *allowed* a release to take place that then carried on down the length of the spine, *allowing* me to lengthen down to the base of my spine and to widen across the pelvis. I suddenly felt solid for the first time and, as a result, I also felt calm and confident. Instead of floundering around in panic it was as if I suddenly had a solid platform to work from for the first time. I was grounded.

Now it was time to work on the throat. Through psycho-physical work I had come to realise what some of my deeper issues were regarding my throat. Not being allowed to express myself and not being heard were some of the key issues from my childhood. So I decided *to give myself permission to speak* and to know that *now was my chance to be heard* regardless of how my audience then reacted to it. I decided at that point to do my best and to let go of the end result. In Alexander terms I stopped being an 'end-gainer'; in psychological terms I had gone beyond any concern about success or failure. I was just going to do my best in the moment regardless of the end result.

Freedom from fear is a big issue. To get to a balanced position I always have to ask myself, "What is the worst thing that can happen?" And if I can face that and realise that I will still be alive and breathing at the end of it, then it can't be so bad. So I consciously went through a list of my worst fears: of appearing stupid, drying up and having nothing to say, everyone laughing at me or people getting up and leaving the room. I consciously went through each one and thought, "And so what, that could happen *but I would still be alive and breathing.*" Suddenly the thought crossed my mind, "Why should I put myself into the victim's position waiting for them to judge me? What do I think of them? What do I want from them?" Suddenly I felt myself getting stronger, as if my energy was beginning to flow out into the world rather than being repressed and held back within myself. I started to feel strong and positive and my mind became clearer. I pursued the line of thinking, looking at the whole situation from the opposite point of view. "They all have to listen to me. I have a captive audience for the next 20 minutes. How wonderful. I know quite a bit about this subject because it is my work and I have researched the material for this talk in great detail. Actually none of the people in this audience know as much as I do. I can visualise them as little children and I am the teacher." I was beginning to feel much more powerful.

I gave directions to *allow* the jaw to release forwards. I also gave directions to *allow* my throat to lengthen into a full contact with my chest, and to *allow* my chest to lengthen into a full contact with my stomach. I felt the tension in my jaw releasing; my breathing was flowing calmly and I heard (as I hummed quietly to myself) how my voice would now be supported by my breathing and resonate from the stomach.

When it came to giving the presentation this time I suddenly felt very confident. Mentally I had decided that even if it all ended in disaster I didn't care, because at least I would have had the satisfaction of knowing that I had played my best shot. So the fear was gone and my energy was moving forwards positively. Using all my knowledge of the Alexander Technique I made sure that I was standing in a well-supported position. Using the lunge position meant that I felt well-grounded and centred in my wide, spacious pelvis. I could feel my heels really drilling into the floor, and my breathing was flowing easily. Maintaining the primary control through the use of directions gave me a sensation of being 'up' and a feeling of really solid presence in the room. Most importantly it slowed down the adrenalin rush so that I was no longer speeding, and my perception of time became more realistic.

One of the most important things I have learnt from the Alexander Technique has been how to *allow* the breath to flow rather than to force it. This links up to the importance of timing when giving a speech on stage or when giving a presentation. There are natural pauses in a text or presentation, where something important has been said and you want the message to sink in. Previously, a pause of several seconds had seemed an eternity of time. I didn't want to appear stupid or as if I had forgotten what I wanted to say. So the tendency had been to rush and to lose audience interest because I appeared to be anxious and going too fast. Now, when I said something important and I wanted the message to sink in I found I had the courage to allow a pause at the appropriate moment, to give the message, "Think about it!" During that pause I found the time to practise my Alexander breathing. This meant that I made sure I had exhaled fully, then I *allowed* the breath to flow in by itself without any sense of effort until the lungs were comfortably full. This took about 10 seconds, but I was giving my audience time to think about what I had just said, and I was giving myself time to recharge from within. By paying attention as I *allowed the breath to flow in* I could check to see if my stomach muscles and the intercostal muscles of my ribcage were relaxed. Through that quality of attention I was calming and centring myself. At the end of that pause I found that I had contacted a power that radiated out from my centre and in some strange magnetic way was able to hold the attention of the other people in the room. The audience seemed to be totally fascinated by what I was saying, but I hadn't been saying anything! I felt that there was a calmness and strength that emanated out from my centre. It was a power that seemed to go beyond words.

After that I was filled with a new sense of confidence that seemed timeless and strangely reassuring. I felt in tune with my audience, and when it came to question time I answered the questions competently without feeling threatened and without feeling that I was trying to prove myself right. There was a sense of a group purpose. Common ground had emerged and the questions that came up were the questions that needed to be looked at and answered for our common benefit.

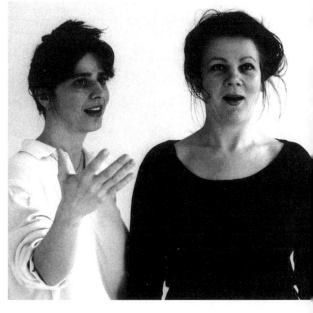

Free your Voice

Let your voice, the tone of your being, flow freely into the world.

Traditionally the benefits of the Alexander Technique have been most appreciated in the performing arts. Actors, musicians, dancers, public speakers have all found the Alexander Technique to be indispensable to their professional skills. Indeed there is hardly a music academy or drama school in the country that does not have an Alexander Technique teacher on its staff helping to train the students. There is always going to be an adrenalin rush and a small (or large!) amount of nervousness just before making an entrance onto the stage. This is part of the nature of public appearances and it adds an important energy to the performance. But it soon wears off as the experienced performer immerses themselves in the role that they are playing. The Alexander Technique is invaluable in that it can prevent stress and nervousness from unnecessarily tightening the voice and breathing, or the smooth action of the arms and fingers as they play a musical instrument, and thus ruining a promising performance.

More than that, on a positive artistic level, the Alexander Technique enhances creativity. When the energy is withdrawn from unnecessary muscular tension into the spine and brain, your intuition becomes heightened and your mind works smoothly and calmly, untroubled by the usual restlessness and anxiety of trivial, everyday concerns. There is a flow of uninterrupted awareness combined with heightened sensitivity that is just brilliant for the creative process. Musicians find that they are able to attune themselves to the flow of a musical composition. Actors are better able to seamlessly take on the character role that they have been assigned. Artists find that they are able to bring some artistic creation to a satisfactory completion, perhaps after an intensely frustrating period of feeling out of tune and blocked.

Where the Alexander Technique has potentially some of its greatest benefits to offer is in the world of professional sport. It has not been fully utilised up till now - possibly due to a mistaken understanding of what terms like 'inhibition' or not being an 'end-gainer' mean. There is nothing wrong in Alexander terms with doing the best you can *in the present moment. Why shouldn't you play your part to the absolute best of your abilities?* There is a lot to be lost by focusing entirely on the end result - which could be worth millions and is therefore very distracting. On top of that, in team sports, there is the added burden psychologically of going out with all the fervent expectations of your team's supporters, or even your country, on top of your shoulders, which again, understandably, can cause you to stiffen up and perform worse rather than better. So purely on the stress prevention level, the Alexander Technique could be very useful.

At the very top level of any sport there is actually very little to distinguish between the technical ability of the top athletes or the top players. They have all had excellent coaching and hours upon hours of training - trained virtually to the level of physical breakdown. The emphasis is on will-power and sheer physical strength and fitness. But as we have discussed in this book earlier on, there are limits as to where the rational intellectual mind and purely physical strength can take you. There comes a level where you need to learn how to 'go with the flow', how to let the inner flow of energy do the work for you rather than trying harder and using even more muscular effort - which is bound to backfire because it will be uncoordinated effort once you reach the limits of your endurance. Go with the flow. It is all about achieving more by doing less.

Everyone has had those occasional experiences of when you hit a shot that just flies away with a satisfying, solid sound. Perfect swing, perfect balance and an unhurried, focused mind. The rhythm of the body movement was perfect so that the body weight goes into the shot rather than pulling back or slightly to the side, and the pivot of the movement is always around the central axis of the spinal column. With that rhythm and balance and *the perfect, focused awareness of the mind in the moment* all the preconditions of the Alexander Technique have been met and there is a free flow of energy, of 'directions', through the body and into the shot.

Tennis players know when they are 'in the zone'; golf players know when their swing is just completely effortless; footballers and cricketers know when their game is just flowing and they seem to have that extra time to be able to read the game and pick out the ball earlier. Athletes know when they have an effortless ease of movement and a lightness that carries them from within. This is all energy flow which, as we know, can be replenished and directed through the body by thought projections or 'directions'. Forget drugs, this is 10 times more powerful. The Alexander Technique does not mean that you have to be inactive and 'inhibit' in order to use it. Quite the contrary, the Alexander Technique is used to tune up your body so that when you go into action there is perfect ease and flow of activity throughout the whole system. A few coaches and players have woken up to the potential benefits of the Technique, and more will follow once the secret is out.

Obviously the one really vital factor that separates out the top teams and the top players is their mental attitude. It is the ability to stay focused and to stay positive even when they are down and things are temporarily not going their way. When playing a tough opponent or when in a tough competition there are bound to be discouraging moments. That is when it is vitally important that negative buttons are not pressed, so that the self-talk stays positive rather than negative. This is doubly important for athletes and sportsmen/women because, as we are psycho-physical beings, a negative mental attitude is immediately reflected in the body posture and patterns of muscular tension, which then affects coordination and performance. It is imperative to be able to spot this happening and to stop it immediately. It isn't enough to just tell yourself, "Be positive, be positive," or, "Focus, focus," or whatever the little phrase is that your coach has taught you. Some of these psychological patterns go deep and it needs the privacy and confidentiality of one-to-one sessions with an Alexander Technique teacher who has also been trained in the subtle technique of psycho-physical rebalancing.

The importance of psycho-physical rebalancing, as explained in the earlier chapter, is that your body wisdom not only helps you to define the root of the problem (which may go all the way back into your childhood), but it also provides the positive antidote and shows the way forwards. Exactly what is preventing you from reaching your full potential? Do you tend to blow it and underperform when you have a big chance? Is there an internal saboteur at work? If there is a fairly consistent pattern of underachievement, then the psychological side needs sorting out in order to free up a more buoyant and consistent performance. This is a totally new psycho-physical pattern that involves both muscular release and a new, more positive mental and emotional attitude. A personal, tailor-made affirmation is provided by your inner body wisdom which can be repeated in times of stress or crisis in order to recall the experience of the new pattern. There is then a solid, calm centre within the body on which to base a positive mental and emotional attitude. Now when you tell yourself to be positive the whole of your bodily experience is supporting that new attitude and it is an inner reality and not just an idea. Some coaches and players already have realised the benefits of incorporating the Alexander Technique into their training preparations, and are able to reap the rewards that this brings them.

Another area where the Alexander Technique is of absolutely fundamental importance is in the sphere of education. It is a long time since I was last at school but the memory of the fear and muscular cramping induced by trying to get it right and trying to please narrow-minded teachers, who were themselves the fear-filled products of a system of educational mass production, remains. I was left with a legacy of feeling stupid and incompetent - even though I made it all the way through primary school, secondary school and university. I emerged with an upper second degree in Economics from a system that totally failed to arouse my interest or engage my creative thinking processes. No wonder I was then left with an aversion to learning anything new - apart from Tai Chi, the Alexander Technique and meditation, which all appeared to be refreshingly anti-intellectual in their approach.

It has taken me a long time to realise that it is not a question of being pro or anti an intellectual educational system; there is a balanced place that incorporates both polarities and then transcends them. That balanced place has to include the totality of the whole human being, the psycho-physical reality of each unique person. Learning, at whatever level, is just the progressive unfoldment of your inner potential. Each person is endowed with infinite inner potential. It is just a question of giving them the time and space to unfold into the world, and the Alexander Technique is the ideal instrument for creating that non-interfering attitude. Learning is always a journey from the known to the unknown. The known is safe and familiar and the unknown can appear strange and frightening, or it can be new and exciting. But this journey necessitates both a willingness to make mistakes and the ability to profit from those mistakes. It is not a question of always getting it right, and there are no 'mistakes' because it is actually a win-win situation; getting it wrong just shows you that this is the wrong route to be following, and therefore it is useful information. You have learnt something useful, so it was not a waste of time at all.

Learning about computers is one example. Young children seem to learn quicker about computers than older adults because they are not afraid to make mistakes - they just try things out and see what happens. Wonderful, the worst thing that can happen is just that the whole computer will crash and you lose your piece of work if you haven't saved it, in which case you restart the computer and have another go. No problem for kids, but quite a big problem for adults. So many adults have negative tapes going in their heads that cause a fearful and contorted posture, and self-blame for being stupid and incompetent when things go wrong. Others develop conspiracy theories about all computers, and their own in particular, being out to sabotage their efforts. It is so interesting to observe your learning process when you first learn something new and potentially difficult.

Obviously what is important in any new enterprise is to connect with your energy and enthusiasm. Why are you learning this? How is it going to help you? What is your motivation? This needs looking at and reassessing as the project develops and as you develop. The same learning task can be done willingly or under threat and duress and it makes a huge difference what your motivation is. As we are free human beings, the more practice we can get at finding the point of freedom, and working with the self-motivating energy that flows from that point, the easier life becomes. The more that energy flows, the more effortless it seems to be to learn or to work, because motivation is the key factor.

Generally in western society, at school, at college and at work, we are taught to equate 'working harder' with a tense and striving attitude. You can see how people grit their teeth, stiffen their necks and tighten muscles throughout their body in an effort to prove to their teacher or boss that they are trying hard. This attitude is carried over subconsciously into all learning situations in later life and it blocks interest, enthusiasm and creative thinking. When learning something new, it is important first of all to face your fear. Fear is the great destroyer, but it operates most powerfully in the darkness of your subconscious processes. As soon as you face it and bring it out into the open it will lose its power. "Look fear in the face and it will cease to trouble you." So ask yourself what is the worst thing that could happen, eg, fear of failure, fear of looking stupid, fear of seeming a slow learner. Whatever it is, if you can bring it out into the open and accept it, look at it without trying to change it or to run away from it, then that is the first step towards resolving it. The deeper issues involved might need psycho-physical rebalancing (as outlined in the earlier chapter). Or, you may be in a position to simply look at your worst fears, imagine them coming true, and imagine yourself still alive and breathing at the end of it all. So, is it really that bad, after all?

Then use what you have learnt about the Alexander Technique. Use the balance exercise to fine-tune your balance; use the breathing exercise to calm the breathing and the mind; use directions to free up primary control and get the energy flowing through an integrated and well-supported body/mind; and then, when you have that feeling of mental calmness and focus, just let the energy flow into activity. If you can keep that feeling of calmness in the background of your mind then everything will flow smoothly. Whatever temporary difficulties you might encounter you will always be able to find the solution. Why? Because, in that calmness, in that attunement, you are able to contact your unlimited inner potential which has the answer to every problem. There are no limitations to what you can learn and do. Everyone has musical ability and can learn to sing and to play a musical instrument - even if they think that they are tone deaf. Everyone can learn about computers, everyone is mathematical and has scientific ability. Some obviously start off with greater natural ability than others, but if your mind is set and you use the Alexander Technique you are capable of anything.

One of the key ways in which the Alexander Technique improves your learning abilities is by increasing your attention span. It gives you the ability to put your attention on any subject that you want to and to hold it there for a sustained period of time. When the primary control is working it *allows* the back to lengthen and widen, which means that you are solidly grounded and calmly aware in the present moment. There are no distractions of past and future and the list of urgent things to be done today. No, there is only the present moment of time and this one single idea or problem that you are focusing your mind on. It is obvious that the concentrated power of attention, focused on this one small area, is going to be far more powerful and successful than a restless and dissipated attention. People think that concentration is a purely mental process - what nonsense. *It is a psycho-physical process.* Why isn't this taught in schools instead of trying to cram children full of factual information? One day it will be. If the motivation is there, and you then calmly focus your mind in the required direction, you can achieve whatever you set out to do, but you need that smooth continuity of uninterrupted thought. The Alexander Technique, by showing you how to go beyond the restlessness of the body, and to focus the energy in the spine and the brain, shows you how to achieve a greatly increased attention span.

The other key factor that the Alexander Technique teaches you is awareness of process. Creativity is a process. You cannot force the end result by having a preconceived idea at the start and then rushing out to make it happen. It just won't work, or it can work but it is a very poor result that you achieve from such 'end-gaining' behaviour. Creativity is a leap of faith, a moving from the known to the unknown and finally to a newly created end result, having a vague idea of what you want in the beginning and trusting to your intuitive feel of what is working well, so that the process will get you there in the end. But you had no idea at the beginning what the end result would be. Process is everywhere in life. Giving 'directions' and *allowing* the end result to happen is process. The simple three-step approach involved in psycho-physical rebalancing is process. Learning any new subject is process, not in the sense of learning a whole series of facts and being able to regurgitate them, but in the sense of making that new understanding your own, a part of you. What stimulates your interest and enthusiasm in that new subject? How does it link up to previous experiences or other areas of interest? How does it challenge you and force you to grow and develop yourself? What intuitions are sparked off, what ideas start to flow from within as you start to play around with these new concepts and ideas? Educate, in its Latin root, comes from *ducere* which means 'to lead', and *educare* means literally 'to lead out' that which is within. It is our unlimited inner potential, which already has all the answers and all the knowledge that we need inside, which needs to be led out into contact with the concepts and knowledge of our society at this present stage of human evolution. How can this process take place through force and coercion? It is a dialogue that can only take place through non-interference and *allowing* for which the Alexander Technique is ideally suited.

If you look at life as an uninterrupted process of learning and self-development then you can see how fundamentally important it is that we learn how to learn properly. Many people are complaining about the pace of change. In this technological era the pace of development is so fast that nothing can remain static any more and job security in the sense of 'jobs for life' is mostly just a thing of the past. Most professions now include the concept of an ongoing professional development programme, because the knowledge that you trained with will soon be outdated, and in the interests of professional competence and efficiency continual updating is essential. Some people love this; many hate it, because they are looking for a comfortable static position. They do not like accepting the challenges of life, and they are not good at coping with change. There is an understandable inner resistance to this process of ongoing change, but this attitude causes unnecessary stress and tension and it costs companies millions each year due to inefficient and undertrained staff.

Through the Alexander Technique it is possible to look at life from a radically new perspective. This acknowledges that life is all about change and self-improvement. The whole purpose of life is to go on improving and growing, doing things that we thought we could never do before, and getting the satisfaction and sense of self-worth that comes with each new accomplishment. Challenges are great because they give us a chance to grow and to prove to ourselves that something that we originally thought to be impossible is actually possible. Seneca once said, *"It is not because things are difficult that we do not dare; it is because we do not dare that they are difficult."* How right he was! It is through this attitude and through action, that we learn to contact our unlimited inner potential. This is a very humanistic viewpoint, but the Alexander Technique provides the key. It provides the technique whereby you can put this philosophy into practice with a calm, relaxed body, easy breathing and a focused mind. Each day, in some little or big way, you should accomplish something that you never thought possible before.

Wouldn't it be fantastic if this was taught in schools, colleges and universities? Wouldn't it be dynamic if large corporations, instead of bribing their top executives to sell their souls and to work those terribly long hours, held prisoner like birds in a gilded cage, taught this inner technique to their employees so that work would be seen as part of a meaningful, balanced existence and an opportunity for true inner satisfaction and self-mastery?

The full implications of the Alexander Technique in the field of education, coping with change and increased job satisfaction have not yet been realised. We are only scratching the surface at the moment. Hopefully the publication of this book (and others), which aims to explain the truly psycho-physical nature of the Alexander Technique in clearly understandable language, will lead to a more widespread use of this wonderful Technique.

One of the greatest psychological challenges people face today is how to increase their sense of self-worth. This is actually a very deep issue with profound implications. There are whole books, whole libraries of self-help manuals that are written about this subject. So many people are suffering from an inner sense of emptiness and worthlessness, desperate for a little bit of love, a little bit of satisfaction. They will go around putting on a surface act, trying to 'be someone', posing, and yet inside there is that inner emptiness, fear and uncertainty. It's tragic; it's such a waste, because most people are looking in the wrong place. You will never find the satisfaction and sense of security that you so desperately want on the outside, in outer possessions or in outer achievements. Never. You will only find it by going deeper within. The answer can only come from the inner solidity and calmness that comes from within as the whole psycho-physical organism changes.

Obviously if there has been a past history of physical, sexual or emotional abuse, this can have devastating consequences for the sense of self-worth in later life. Painful though it is, these issues have to be faced and dealt with first of all before any real progress can be made with improving the sense of self-worth. The technique of psycho-physical rebalancing that has already been outlined (in Chapter 8) is an ideal technique for resolving issues of abuse. It gets to the truth of the experience that has been stored as a trauma in the body memory of the client, *and to what that experience meant for the client.* The work can be graduated and taken at a manageable pace. Most importantly, through psycho-physical rebalancing, the client is able to leave the session in a balanced and together state. I have been able to deal successfully with abuse issues through the technique of psycho-physical rebalancing, though it is obviously long-term work that requires serious commitment on both sides.

Having dealt with any major issues that may be related to earlier experiences of abuse, it is then possible to *allow* the whole psycho-physical organism to stay grounded, open and receptive to the ever-present flow of life energy. Everything that has been written in this book about adopting a more positive and supportive body language through the use of balance, breathing, directions and maintaining mental calmness applies. As the Alexander Technique is a psycho-physical technique you gradually come to realise that this improved body posture actually leads to a different mental attitude and a different energy flow throughout the body. This will then attract different experiences and relationships into your life. Of the greatest importance is the ability to remain properly grounded in the pelvis. From this centre it is possible to ask yourself what you want and what you need in any given situation and thus counteract any tendency to feel abused or imposed on by more powerful personalities at work or at home. You might not always be able to get what you want but you can at least ask for it, and having verbalised it you are then in a position to negotiate and may well end up getting 50 per cent. Even if you get nothing because the other side is too powerful or intractable you have at least had the satisfaction of saying what you need and verbalising your position instead of holding back - which a lot of people with low self-esteem do.

Due to an improved, more confident body language you are far more likely to meet with a positive response from the world, whilst a collapsed, apologetic posture is inviting rejection. You may also find that due to the Alexander Technique you have a lot more energy, resulting both from better posture and also from being more in touch with your real needs and genuine enthusiasm for life. As you come into contact with this increased energy flow, and maintain the primary control, you will find that you can initiate more projects, work more productively and achieve more in the course of a day. All in a relaxed, almost nonchalant manner. It's called 'being in the flow'. As a result of this, more gets achieved and therefore your sense of self-esteem goes up, because self-worth is undoubtedly related to what you are able to achieve in your life. Don't get me wrong, it's not because of the increased power or position or earning capacity. It is nothing to do with those external things; that is merely secondary and only of significance insofar as it helps you to fulfil your responsibilities and to help others. The real significance comes from the inner sense of accomplishment, of having visualised a goal, made an effort, overcome all difficulties and having finally brought things to a successful conclusion. That is what starts to build up your self-esteem, and each little victory is cumulative.

But it goes deeper than this; it goes right to the core. At the third stage of the Alexander Technique you realise that with the increase in the power of the flow you have become different from what you were before. You may suddenly realise that the power flowing into you is not the product of your will but comes from somewhere else, and that all you have to do is to keep the primary control open, let in that flow of energy, and use it positively. There is then a joyous realisation that that power is the power of Life, the power of the Cosmos, the Greater Whole (call it what you will) flowing through you. You have become an open and willing channel for the Cosmos to work through. As you simply fulfil each of your life's duties in a willing and receptive mode, this results in a transformation, a deepening of the meaning and content of every situation as well as the power to fulfil all of your responsibilities and overcome difficulties. And thus everything acquires a new perspective. If you just answer the call of each duty with an accepting and enthusiastic attitude to the best of your ability, obstacles will mysteriously clear from your path, one thing will lead to another and you will ultimately be led towards the task that is your life purpose and the fulfilment of your life's destiny. You will find that you are doing what you are meant to be doing, effortlessly. You are then way beyond any question of having a low or high self-esteem, you are just doing what you have to be doing irrespective of other people's opinions. You are playing your role on the stage of life perfectly and to the best of your abilities, and enjoying it.

Chapter 10

THE SPIRITUAL DIMENSION OF THE ALEXANDER TECHNIQUE

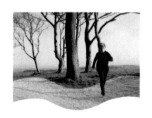

Who am I? What is the purpose of my existence here? Where have I come from and where am I going to? These are the great spiritual questions that everyone will have to ask themselves at some point in their lives, even if it is only a fearful wondering at the point of death. Is there an afterlife or is death the cessation of all consciousness? The Egyptians certainly believed in life after death. Numerous scenes painted on papyrus scrolls show the dead being led into the Hall of Judgement by the jackal-headed god, Annubis. There, the heart is placed on the scales of judgement and balanced against a feather of truth. If the heart is heavy with sin and deceit, it will outweigh the feather, and that person will not be able to enter the joyous afterlife, and the heart will be devoured by Ammit the devourer. If the life has been pure, Horus will present the soul of that person to the radiant Osiris, the god of the underworld. There are no secrets from the gods in the Hall of Judgement. The Hindu and Buddhist traditions speak of the Law of Karma, which says that you reap what you sow and that all your good or evil thoughts and actions will inevitably come back to you as the circle is completed. You only harm yourself when you harm someone else, and you are doing yourself a favour when you help someone else.

The Alexander Technique itself has no moral framework or spiritual perspective and keeps itself safely distanced from such complex questions. However, Alexander would certainly agree that our thoughts and actions have consequences that come back to us in the fullness of time. We do have freedom of choice and yet it is not absolute freedom, because we are bound by the consequences of our actions. This is where Alexander's concept of reaching a point of freedom where you are able to calmly decide what your best option is becomes of crucial importance. A rushed decision is never a good decision. If you are too lazy to think what the consequences of any given action might be, then you will have to experience them directly later on, and the consequences might be very unpleasant. That is not totally negative because you might even learn a positive lesson from the experience, but the unthinking habitual repetition of a damaging habit pattern just because something feels 'right' (through the power of repetition) and enjoyable is foolish and just leads to ultimate misery.

This is where Alexander's concept of pausing for a period of time ('inhibition') becomes of crucial importance. You can get in tune by giving directions and remaining in a place of creative indifference *until you are certain that you have contacted your inner intuitive guidance and are doing the right thing.* It is more than sage advice to think carefully before you act. The practice of the Alexander Technique actually enables you to get in touch with your higher self, or your soul intuition, so that your actions become wisdom-guided actions rather than impulsive decisions that are determined by habit and short-term gratification. This concept of spiritualising your thinking, and acting in tune with your higher wisdom for the highest good of yourself and others, is of fundamental importance if you want to make any progress on the spiritual path. It is at the heart of all moral injunctions and spiritual discipline. Each person is unique with a unique character and ingrained habit patterns. It takes constant vigilance and self-observation in order to be able to change your character for the better. It is of little use just reading spiritual books that describe what the ideal state is like. You have to start with your unique character and where you are at this moment in time. Then you need constant individual guidance

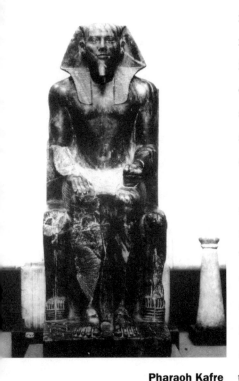

Pharaoh Kafre

He certainly knew how to sit well, and this sculpture would suggest that he also knew how to meditate deeply.

in dealing with situations and overcoming negative habit patterns. This can only come from your own higher wisdom. And the practice of the Alexander Technique, by refining your sensitivity and awareness of that inner intuitive spiritual guidance, helps you to keep progressing on the spiritual path.

Correct posture and a strong flow of life energy along the spine is the basic foundation on which any successful meditation practice must be based. The practice of some form of meditation or 'stillness' is essential if you want to find God and achieve spiritual liberation. You cannot sit and meditate successfully with a crooked spine. It cannot be done. The foundation of any meditation technique is correct posture. In traditional spiritual training, maintaining good posture - the correct *asana* of meditation - was recognised as the basis of all further practices. In Zen monasteries a senior monk would tour the meditation halls with a big bamboo stick ready to deliver a sharp reminder to any novice who had allowed their posture to collapse or who had gone to sleep! A harsh practice that is unsuited to a more indulgent age. Anyway, you can attain the same results quicker and more easily through spending a few minutes practising the Alexander Technique at the start of your meditation period. The ancient Egyptians certainly knew how to meditate, sitting beautifully balanced on a chair, as you can see from numerous sculptures in their temples. The Hindu and the Buddhist traditions tend to stress sitting on the floor in a full or half-lotus position, but the only essential factor is to have a strong, balanced posture where the energy can flow up along a free spine.

It is the subtlety of the indirect approach and 'non-doing' that makes the Alexander Technique such a good foundation on which to build any system of spiritual discipline and meditation. It is impossible to force results to satisfy the ego through the use of will-power and muscular straining. It cannot succeed; you will never get any valid results either in the Alexander Technique or in meditation through these sorts of methods. Both Alexander Technique and meditation share the same central paradox: you cannot achieve your goal by trying, but only by 'non-doing' and detachment. Results, when they come, come in their own time as a result of transcending the ego, creating space, and allowing the energy to flow through you, not through making the ego stronger by the practice of strenuous ascetic disciplines that you can use to impress others and to boast about. There is the constant danger of 'spiritual materialism' in any sort of spiritual practice. Questions like, "What have I got out of it? How many spiritual experiences have I had? How far have I advanced? How far have they advanced?" are all indications of egotism and a spiritual 'end-gaining' attitude that is causing tension and blocking any further progress. When you base your spiritual practice upon the foundation of the Alexander Technique instead and just pay attention to your posture and the free flow of energy along the spine, you can be in the moment without any expectation of results. Give up striving, give up looking for results and create a space where God can enter. The results will then come by themselves when you create a vacuum by overcoming the ego, and you will be pleasantly surprised at how effective your spiritual practice can be. You need constant practice of your spiritual techniques - simple though they may be - *the practice is the point* not the results. Because through repeated practice you are not going anywhere but you are overcoming the ego and remaining exactly where you are in the present moment of time but with a heightened state of consciousness. This attitude is what the Alexander Technique can contribute in its highest essence.

As the energy moves up and down the spine it starts the circulation of light that in time will energise and illumine each of the seven chakras. These are petals of light that are visible to the inner vision, lined up along the spine from the earth chakra at the base of the spine, right up to the thousand-petalled lotus of divine bliss situated on the crown of the head. The circulation is originally around the first six chakras until sufficient voltage of current has built up to illumine the seventh crown chakra, which then glows with light and joy, like the halo around the head of a saint. The directions 'forward and up' in the Alexander Technique curve the energy in a forward arc to the 'third eye' between the eyebrows (otherwise known as the spiritual eye, the star of the East or the eye of Horus). This is the sixth chakra and it is the only chakra that has two sides to it: the back side at the medulla oblongata, where the brain stem tapers off into the spinal column, which controls the inflow of life energy into the body (Alexander called this the 'primary control'); and the front side at the point between the eyebrows, which is the centre of our creative visualisation, spiritual thinking, spiritual will and telepathic thought, which Alexander called the 'forward and up'. There is a natural flow of energy along the spine once a positive pole has been established at the third eye and a negative pole has been established at the base of the spine, at the root chakra, through proper grounding. Even a little practice at keeping this flow of energy going whilst concentrating at the third eye brings a feeling of great peace, love and joy. The point of meditation is to become one with that, to melt into that, so that you can affirm and feel, *I am this river of peace and love and joy.* It is also possible to see the third eye during deep meditation. This appears at first as a sensation of light, which clarifies into two outstretched golden wings (hence the 'dove of light' in the Bible, or the Egyptian Hawk God) which then sharpen into a clear visual perception of three concentric circles. The outer circle is gold, the middle circle is dark blue and the innermost circle is like being drawn into a rotating dark tunnel that has an incredibly beautiful five-pointed white star at the end of it. There is a feeling of upliftment and expansion of consciousness. If you can stay calmly concentrated on this point it is possible to start moving down the tunnel towards the five-pointed white star.

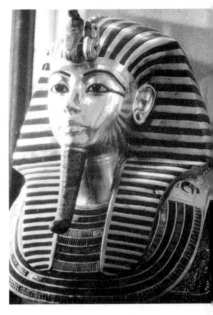

Gold Death Mask of Pharaoh Tutankhamen

This shows the hooded cobra emerging from the third eye in the forehead between the eyebrows.

This is the single eye of Horus, depicted in so many Egyptian paintings and manuscripts, and the tunnel is the doorway to the spiritual realms. In the New Testament it says, "If, therefore, thine eye be single, thy whole body shall be full of light." To many biblical scholars this has always seemed a meaningless phrase, probably due to a mistranslation, which they could not understand. Actually the translation is accurate and it refers to the deepest spiritual truth - that in the deep calmness of meditation the glow of the single spiritual eye will appear. The Egyptian Pharaohs were often sculpted with the image of a hooded cobra coming out of their foreheads at this point. This is symbolic of the whole energy flow, from the coiled serpent-like passageway in the earth chakra at the root of the spine, where the energy flow is awakened, right up to the light of the spiritual eye at the sixth chakra. The symbolism has remained the same in different cultures, eg, the Hindu technique of Kundalini Yoga refers to exactly the same process.

Although the Alexander Technique is not a meditation technique in itself, by strengthening the flow of energy through the spine and by following certain key spiritual laws it lays the secure foundation for the successful practice of any spiritual discipline. The teachings of Paramahansa Yogananda, who first brought Kriya Yoga to the West, are explicitly based on the psycho-physical nature of meditation and the movement of energy up and down the spine. Kriya is a very advanced form of meditation and the free flow of energy through the spine is an essential prerequisite for successful practice. The calm, blissful sensation of energy flowing up and down the spine that is felt during an Alexander Technique lesson is greatly amplified during Kriya. Eventually you can learn to see the spiritual eye and, holding the consciousness steady, to pass through the tunnel of the spiritual eye into the astral realm, leaving the body behind. For anyone who has learnt the Alexander Technique and is interested in learning this simple yet powerful meditation technique I can recommend getting in touch with Self-Realization Fellowship in California. (You can find them listed under useful addresses at the back of this book.)

Breath is the bridge between mind and body. In any form of spiritual practice or study you have to be able to calm the breath in order to be able to go deep. If you practise the method of breathing recommended by Alexander you will soon discover that there is a crucial moment at the balance point between the inhalation and exhalation, and between exhalation and inhalation. Each time you breathe in or out there is a fraction of a second, or longer, when you can quite happily remain in a state of breathlessness without any desire to breathe at all. This is not a forced state, it is a very enjoyable and natural cessation of breath. As it says in the Bible, "Man shall not live by bread alone but by every word that proceedeth out of the mouth of God." As well as an invitation to spiritual study, this is a key reference as to how it is possible for man (ie, human beings) to live without breathing, sustained directly by the inflow of cosmic life energy (ie, the 'word') from the 'primary control' at the medulla oblongata (the 'mouth of God'). Correct practice of the Alexander Technique enables you to dramatically slow the breath, and even to exist quite comfortably for short periods of time without any desire or need of breathing. In that calmness and inner stillness it is easier to focus the mind and to keep it focused on any object of thought - which is a prerequisite of any meditation technique.

I have had many students who have used the Alexander method of breathing in order to calm themselves down during stressful periods of the day and as a preparation for meditation. I have also had a few students who have spontaneously seen the third eye (without any suggestion on my part) when practising deep, calm Alexander breathing in the semi-supine position on the table, whilst I was directing the energy flow along the spine. They had a sensation of light, of either gold or dark blue colour, and they reported feeling an upliftment and expansion of consciousness as they stayed calmly concentrated on this point.

Spirit is subtle and intangible. It takes time and constant practice to get in tune with the realm of spirit and then you will gradually realise that the unreal is real and what you thought to be so real (ie, the material universe surrounding us) is actually unreal. Alexander first hinted at this with his concept of 'faulty sensory appreciation' where he showed that what you think is happening in your body is not what is happening at all: it is a total delusion based on the repetition of habits. In the same way, what you perceive to be the reality of the world around you is a delusion based on the repetition of habitual thoughts and assumptions. It is only with time and the practice of the 'primary control' that you are able to get in touch with the accurate sensory appreciation of what is really happening in your body. How does this work? It is your intuitive awareness extending through the energetic flow of 'directions' that actually gives you an accurate idea of what is going on in your body.

Human beings are definitely enmeshed in the cosmic play of *Maya* or cosmic delusion and what is the way out? The key lies in finding a way to transcend habitual thoughts and assumptions and through the law of balance to find the point of freedom and escape. Through mind control and self-awareness it is possible to reach a point of 'creative indifference' where there are no desires and no preferences one way or the other. It is possible to train this by looking at people or objects with total acceptance because that is *what is* that's the way they are right now and there are reasons for it all. I can look at a tree without liking the colour or disliking the shape. I can look at people without allowing myself to be critical or idealising them according to immediate reactions and preferences. I can look at them in full awareness and be non-judgemental of their personal characteristics. When I reach that state of consciousness I am at a balanced place, without the likes or dislikes of the ego, and then God will be sucked in to fill that vacuum by the atmospheric pressure of his omnipresence.

The law of creative indifference is the law of all laws:

Empty yourself and you shall be full.
Accept yourself and you shall be transformed.

This is clearly practised in the Alexander Technique when *allowing* things to happen by giving 'directions' and 'inhibiting' at the same time; it creates a space of creative indifference. This is the basic spiritual law - things come to you when you don't want them any more, eg, with creative ideas, inventions, relationships, business contracts. The crucial breakthrough always comes when you have let go of wanting it. To apply this law does not mean that you enter a totally inactive and passive state. It's not that easy! It means that you apply the principles of creative indifference (perhaps you use the Alexander Technique to help you get into that balanced mental state) and you keep on working at it (or you can take a break while your subconscious mind keeps on working at it) but you are not in a state of mental and emotional tension due to a driving personal desire for results. It is exactly the same principle that Krishna advised Arjuna to adopt in the Bhagavad Gita: do your duty, the things that life is demanding from you every day, to the best of your ability and with full mental awareness,

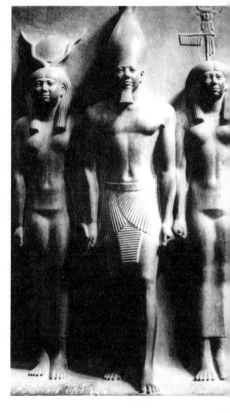

Pharaoh Menkaure with Two Wives

Notice how Menkaure chooses to stand in the stability of the lunge position. The law of creative indifference is illustrated by the symbolism on top of his first wife's head, the circle of spirit rising up between the two prongs of duality.

but without personal preferences or the thought of personal reward at the end of the day. This isn't just a state of passive awareness, it is creative indifference applied to dynamic activity.

Many people wonder why their prayers do not work. It is mostly because they are not obeying this law. *God is limitless: You cannot put a limit on God!* They are praying and they want a definite result, now! But God is beyond all dualities and relativities of manifestation, beyond time and space. So when praying for physical or material help you cannot put a time limit on it. Through God's grace, healing power will flow into you at exactly the right point in time when you need it, and not before! Actually God only exists in the present moment so if you can go beyond your dualistic thinking and connect with that, it has already happened. You just need a direction that can link your present need with that point in (what we call) the future where the perfect answer already exists. But you have to get beyond that delusion of separation and realise that the answer exists right now, in the Here and Now, the eternal present of God's omnipresence.

So the ability to remain firmly grounded in the present moment, in full acceptance of what is happening right now, is crucial. This gives that power of prayer, and it is an attitude that needs to pervade all of life. The whole point of spiritual development is not to have special powers, visions and mystical experiences (although these may come in the fullness of time). It is to remain right where you are in your life and to bear all life's burdens with a resilience and an inner strength. You can do this by channelling and focusing your energies from within. Take the analogy of a mountain torrent that is dammed to create a reservoir. This head of water behind the dam can then be channelled to drive turbines and create useful electricity. It's the same when you learn to control and channel the life force, taking it up and down the spine: it leads to an increase in inner strength and to true spiritual advancement. This helps you in coping with change, maintaining a calm centre as you deal with the inevitable ups and downs of life, dealing with the things that you can change and accepting the things that you can't. *Acceptance: "It doesn't get any better than this! This present moment is all there is and it is perfect, as I attune myself with God's omnipresence it doesn't get better than this."* Keep reminding yourself when the ego comes up with some plan or some desire. Under all circumstances refuse to worry! It doesn't help.

It is hard to do this when life is full of such sudden and unexpected change. The attack on New York and Washington and the destruction of the twin towers of the World Trade Centre, is one shocking example. Thousands of innocent lives were lost on September 11th, 2001. This clearly is the start of a dramatic period in world history. My only advice, which is being repeated by America's allies, is not to overreact in an habitual manner. More killing of thousands of innocent people, which cannot be hidden from our TV screens, will not make the world situation any better, it will just add to the snowball of negative karma that already exists. The guilty should be punished, but it is wrong for more innocent people to be killed. But decisions like this are outside of my sphere of influence, so all I can do is to remain true to my own spiritual principles, practise the Alexander Technique, and meditate; whilst remaining in the flow and doing whatever good I can do in my own immediate environment. I know from the Alexander Technique and my spiritual principles that the most important thing is to stay calm, pause for a while and then do the right thing. Obviously there has to be some form of reaction, but everything has a reason and it is part of a great universal plan. There is good in bad and bad in good. Some possible good that could come from this is the creation of a global police force with the power to track down international terrorists. There could also be a trend towards more decentralisation with people working from smaller offices in the countryside, linked by computers. We are witnessing the gradual breakdown of outer authority structures, and we are living in a period of accelerating change. The only answer is to look within and to find your own inner authority structure, your inner spiritual compass, that will tell you what is right or wrong. At the end of the day the only person you can change is yourself, and the only real contribution you can make to the world is to change yourself for the better.

Global warming is another slowly ticking time bomb. Already the Gulf Stream has decreased by 20 per cent with a significant impact on the European climate. The Pacific El Niño current has also changed. As global warming accelerates and we have to face the huge ecological and climatic changes triggered off by man-made pollution and the melting ice caps we will all need a technique that can increase spiritual protection whilst we remain inwardly calm and centred. Grounded in the inner security of unshakeable inner convictions, we must do what we can in our own local situations. More people could go back to the land and live simply, growing their own vegetables and living in spiritual communities. There is nothing to do except to surrender to the inevitable as the planet moves on to a new stable equilibrium point with a repositioning of the polar axis (no one can be sure where). This is an example of the principles of transformation and rebalancing on a global scale and, as you apply the principles of self-transformation in your own life, changing yourself for the better, you are aiding the planet in its evolutionary process. The immanence of change, suddenly feeling threatened and vulnerable - this all raises questions in people's minds and many more will turn to religion or some system of spiritual development for inner support. As Paramahansa Yogananda said, we will have to learn to, "Stand unshaken midst the crash of breaking worlds."

THE IMPORTANCE OF BALANCE

Balance is the key to the Alexander Technique and unless we can broaden our understanding to include the concept of a living balance, and what this means in practice, we will never quite get the hang of the Technique.

Balance means to live in the tension of the opposites and to enjoy the freedom existing at the fulcrum, the central point where two opposing forces counterbalance in exact equality and opposition to each other. It is similar to the calm existing in the eye of the hurricane. If we look at the universe we can see how balance is actually playing a pivotal role in keeping the whole system unified. Take our solar system for example, where the earth is orbiting the sun, completing one revolution in a year. There are obviously two forces at work: one is the centrifugal force of the earth's orbit that threatens to send us spinning off into outer space; and the other is the gravitational pull of the sun which threatens to pull us into its fiery heart. This force varies directly, as the product of the masses, and inversely, as the square of the distance the earth and the sun are apart. Yet the orbit of the earth traces out precisely that path where these two forces are balanced out, and up until now no stray comet

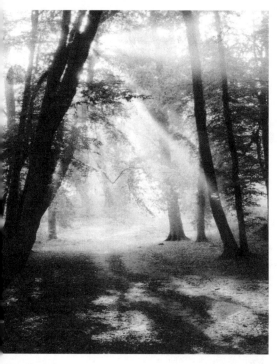

Woodland Light

Energy flows up the trunk towards the crown of the tree as the light streams downwards.

or meteorite has hit us with sufficient force to knock us out of orbit and send us spinning off to our doom. Isn't that wonderful? It is the same when we stand on the earth. There is the force of gravity linking our centre with the centre of the earth, and yet at that point where our feet touch the ground the thrust of our body weight downwards calls forth an equal and opposite reaction from the earth, so that there is in fact a counter-thrust, an anti-gravitational force, if you like, that travels upwards through our body to the crown of our head. This is what enables us to keep our balance and maintain an upright posture. Curiously enough most people do not allow themselves to feel this counter-thrust because they are so busy contracting themselves, tensing muscles and pulling inwards, instead of relaxing, lengthening their muscles and allowing the play of these forces throughout their skeletal and muscular systems. It could all be so easy and natural if we were just calmly aware of what is happening within us.

Everybody living on the material plane is struggling with the problem of polarity. Light and shadow, pleasure and pain, ease and disease - the list is endless if you analyse it. All our problems stem from the fact that we are adopting an extreme position, and pinning our hopes of happiness upon attaining one extreme and holding onto it for as long as possible. Alexander called such people 'end-gainers', and he was highly suspicious of this attitude. Experience and introspection had shown him that he had exhibited a strong tendency in this respect, and the futility of such an attitude had become fully apparent to him.

There is a spiritual dimension to balance, which is beautifully illustrated by the old Chinese Yin/Yang symbol. One half is white and the other half is black, symbolising the duality of experience inherent on this material plane. The nature of our mind is such that we seem always to be chasing after one polarity and attempting to negate the existence of the other, the basis of our assumption being that if we can just gain our objective and hold onto it for long enough, our happiness will be assured. However, as most of us have come to realise - usually as a result of great pain and disillusionment - life simply isn't like that. The Yin exists only as a contrast to the Yang, and vice versa: neither can exist independently of the other. If we examine the nature of our experiences carefully we will come to see that indeed nothing stays the same for ever. Nothing is permanent; there are always going to be problems; there is always going to be good and bad in a world of duality. Yet there remains in us a powerful urge to grasp and experience some sort of absolute and permanent fulfilment. What is the answer? We know that if we push too far towards one extreme we will reach a point where we begin to pull back towards its opposite. We then make the mistake of believing that some outside force is responsible and we contract into ourselves. We enter 'victim' mode and, whether we like to admit it or not, this is perfectly reflected in our body posture, visible for all to see.

What then is the answer? A clear recognition and acceptance that as long as we identify totally with our bodies, ie, one extreme of a polarity, believing that we are a law unto ourselves, able to do whatever we want and to satisfy all our desires instantaneously, we are caught in this interplay of opposites and there is no escaping it. This is law. No amount of denial will change it. Ultimately, sufficient experience of being hurt and disappointed usually spurs us on to search for deeper meaning in our lives, and perhaps we join a church or become involved in a system of spiritual teaching where we hope - certainly in the beginning (if we are honest enough to admit it!) - that God or our teaching will provide us with some magical power to bring about the fulfilment of our old desires and wishes. We may at some stage pass through a period in which we try to negate our physical aspect altogether, attempting now to assume a purely 'spiritual' identity. However, we are still left with bodies on this earth and before long we find we are trapped in yet another bid to cling to an extreme. It is not, therefore, until we begin to realise that, contrary to our belief thus far, the answer to our dilemma lies in ceasing to strive to be anything: that we do not exist separately from God, Life, the Flow - call it what you will - and that the 'personality', limited by body and matter, the poor little victim at sea in an ocean of change, needs merely to undergo a shift of identity. We are the Flow. Our individual consciousness might be described as a unique facet or window through which this Flow may pour forth into manifestation. And so the purpose of practising the Alexander Technique may be summed up as a means of focusing and becoming conscious of our true centre, enabling us to identify fully and willingly with that equipoise which is absolute stillness, and from which the extraordinary dynamic of polarity issues as effect.

We remain, however, at all times, rooted in cause, and we flower as effect. Balance. No further need to grasp or to become. Now we can simply relax and be.

It might seem strange to say but if we study the Yin/Yang symbol we may discover that the most important thing about it is actually the relationship between the two poles. Draw a line from any point on the circumference through the centre and out to the opposite point, and you will find that there are exactly equal portions of black and white along the length of the diameter. Surprising? Not really. There is always perfect balance and harmony in this symbol. And if we view it as a guide to apply to our experiences in life, its message becomes obvious: don't try to fix, hold, or waste your time trying to identify yourself more fully with one or the other portion. Accept what comes to you, and remain even-minded. By remaining centred we allow a natural harmony to resonate between the pairs of opposites, thus freeing ourselves from the compulsion to make judgements and comparisons of any kind. The Alexander Technique provides one of the most practical and understandable methods for applying these principles in day-to-day living, for one notices a transformation in one's life almost immediately.

Looked at in this light, many of the oft-posed questions about life, its purpose, one's destiny, and so on, lose their pertinence, because life is seen more and more as a great balancing act wherein one's experiences need not be taken too seriously. Why? Because a shift in our identity is beginning to take place, and we recognise that outer experiences do not have the power to touch our true essence. Perfectly poised within the profound stillness at the 'eye of the hurricane', we can allow the play of duality to dance around us. True freedom always lies at the centre, at that balance point, and you could even say that the balance point between these two apparently irreconcilable opposites of spirit and matter is human consciousness, as it becomes progressively aware of spirit working creatively in matter, and matter transforming itself back into the consciousness of spirit again.

USEFUL CONTACT ADDRESSES

If you are interested in training courses or individual sessions with me, Alex Maunder, in Psycho-Physical Rebalancing or the Alexander Technique please look for details on my website at:

www.alexandy.dircon.co.uk

Corporate training details are on: re-sourcing.co.uk

If you wish to contact an Alexander Technique teacher in your area please write to:

The Society of Teachers of the Alexander Technique
129 Camden Mews
London NW1 9AH
Tel: 020 7284 3338

or log on to the STAT website at: www.stat.org.uk

Meditation techniques and Kriya Yoga, as taught by Paramahansa Yogananda, can be learnt from Self-Realization Fellowship at:

SRF International Headquarters
3880 San Rafael Avenue
CA 90065-3298
USA
Tel: (001) 323 225 2471

Website: www.yogananda-srf.org

BIBLIOGRAPHY

FM Alexander,
Man's Supreme Inheritance
Centerline Press, 1988.

FM Alexander,
*The Universal Constant
in Living*
Centerline Press, 1986.

FM Alexander,
*Constructive Conscious
Control of the Individual*
Centerline Press, 1985.

FM Alexander,
The Use of the Self
Centerline Press, 1984.

Walter Carrington,
The Act of Living
Mornum Time Press, 1999.

Petruska Clarkson,
Gestalt Counselling in Action
Sage Publications, 1992.

Jonathan Drake,
Body Know-How
Thorsons, 1991.

Karlfried Graf von Durkheim,
Hara
Otto Wilhelm Barth Verlag, 1987.

Viktor Frankl,
Man's Search for Meaning
Washington Square Press, 1959.

Michael Gelb,
Body Learning
Aurum Press, 1981.

Eugene Gendlin,
Focusing
Bantam Books, 1979.

Stanley Kellerman,
Somatic Reality
Center Press, 1979.

James Kepner,
Body Process
Jossey-Bass Publishers, 1993.

James Kepner,
Healing Tasks
Jossey-Bass Publishers, 1995.

Alexander Lowen,
The Language of the Body
Collier Books, 1958.

Perls, Hefferline & Goodman,
Gestalt Therapy
Souvenir Press, 1951.

Candace Pert,
The Molecules of Emotion
Simon & Shuster, 1998.

Debbie Shapiro,
The Bodymind Workbook
Element, 1990.

Paramahansa Yogananda,
Autobiography of a Yogi
Self-Realization Fellowship, 1946.

INDEX